OUT OF THE
SHADOWS

OUT OF THE
SHADOWS

WALLY LEWIS

with Neil Cadigan

HarperSports
An imprint of HarperCollinsPublishers

Harper*Sports*
An imprint of HarperCollins*Publishers*

First published in 2009
This edition published in 2010
by HarperCollins*Publishers* Australia Pty Limited
ABN 36 009 913 517
harpercollins.com.au

HarperCollins*Publishers*
25 Ryde Road, Pymble, Sydney, NSW 2073, Australia
31 View Road, Glenfield, Auckland 0627, New Zealand

National Library of Australia Cataloguing-in-Publication data:

Lewis, Wally, 1959–
    Out of the shadows / Wally Lewis with Neil Cadigan.
    2nd ed.
    ISBN: 978 0 7322 8881 5 (pbk.)
    Lewis, Wally, 1959–
    Rugby League football – Australia – Biography.
    Rugby League football players – Australia – Biography.
    Epileptics – Australia – Biography.
    Other Authors/Contributors: Cadigan, Neil
796.3338092

Cover design: Design by Committee
Front cover photograph by Steve Baccon
Back cover images (from left to right): © Action Photographics, © Action
    Photographics, © Newspix, © Mark Evans/Newspix
Typeset in 11.5/18pt Bembo by Kirby Jones
Printed and bound in Australia by Griffin Press
70gsm Classic used by HarperCollins*Publishers* is a natural, recyclable product
made from wood grown in sustainable forests. The manufacturing processes
conform to the environmental regulations in the country of origin, Finland.

5 4 3 2 1   10 11 12 13

As a small boy I knew little about epilepsy, or the struggle involved. As a man, my understanding of the disease remained minor but, through experience, I became well educated about its effect.

Yet, sadly, it remains one of the world's least promoted medical struggles. It's time to help the millions who remain in the dark — as I've found, there is light at the end of the tunnel.

This book is dedicated to all those affected by epilepsy.

CONTENTS

PREFACE

By Neil Cadigan

WALLY Lewis has never been comfortable with the tag of 'The King', as in the king of State of Origin. However, as 'Origin' football, the modern rugby league phenomenon, passes its 30th season, the validity of the label has not diminished.

His eight man-of-the-match awards is still a record. So too is his eight series wins from 11 as Queensland captain, including the 1981 one-off game (he had 19 victories in 31 matches for the Maroons). A statue of him holding aloft the interstate shield stands proudly outside of Suncorp Stadium (called Lang Park when he kicked a leather ball around the ground in the 1980s) and Queenslanders still bow to it as they pass.

However, Wally Lewis — one of only seven rugby league players officially tagged 'Immortals' — had a love–hate image during his rugby league playing days; with opinion determined by which state you were aligned to.

In Brisbane, 'The Emperor of Lang Park' (a title placed upon him by the Godfather-like figure of Queensland Rugby League, Ron McAuliffe) would have maroon-clad supporters bowing and chanting 'Wally … Wally' as if to hail a messiah of their state. In Sydney, the chant would be extended to 'Wally's a wanker' or 'Wally sucks', as a response to him stealing the Australian captaincy from the almost-exclusive half-century possession by New South Wales favourites, his dominance of Origin man-of-the-match awards (including five from six games in 1982–84), the pedestal he was elevated onto by the Queensland public and media, and a perceived arrogant nature.

That was his split personality; split by the interstate border between Queensland and New South Wales. Even when he captained Australia, which he did so magnificently in 24 of his 34 Tests (1981–91), he could be subject to that interstate jealousy which was as shamefully disrespectful as it was ridiculous. He was once booed by a 'home' crowd in Sydney as the stadium screen captured him while the national anthem played before a Test match, a despicable contempt of patriotism.

In a warped sort of way, it was testimony to his greatness. He was *the* super figure of State of Origin just when it needed a hero, and required Queensland success to establish it in the early 1980s. It seems illogical today that critics had perceived it as a manufactured event created purely to please Queensland egos (how wrong they were).

Like many things in life, hindsight can purify judgement. And it was a heart-warming moment to hear the genuineness of the applause Wally received when introduced, as a member of Australian rugby league's Team of the Century, to the crowd at the Sydney Cricket Ground for the Centenary Test match between Australia and New Zealand in May 2008. By then it had been revealed he suffered epilepsy and had recovered from a major brain operation which has removed seizures from his life.

Wally could command a game of rugby league, almost as a puppeteer, better than any rugby league player over a century, save for Andrew Johns who came along two years after Lewis' last club game for the battling Gold Coast Seagulls. No one in his era could dictate the momentum of a match with such effectiveness as Walter James Lewis. During the 1980s, only Parramatta halfback Peter Sterling, in NSW club football, attracted such 'stop him at all costs' attention in match plans, yet so consistently proved 'ungettable'. Wally epitomised the strong rugby league edict of being the player others wanted to play with; as any of his team-mates will testify.

Yet he alienated people, and shook off that polarisation with a dogged determination to succeed on the football field for whoever he was representing — club, state or country. And he succeeded with such ease, often taking a back seat until the pinnacle moment of a match needed his influence and then he would be unstoppable.

Two matches stand in my memory which typify his ability to impact himself and change a match's direction. One was at Central Park, Wigan, in England on the 1986 Kangaroo tour during which he captained Australia to their second (successive) undefeated tour over 78 years. The Australians were under the pump for the first time in the series as they knew they were one victory away from completing the English leg of the tour unbeaten. The score was 12-all and the Brits were clearly playing better than the tourists. After a bit of push and shove between players, Lewis niggled British prop Chris Burton into a punching frenzy, tempting French referee Julian Rascagneres to sin-bin Burton. Dale Shearer scored a penalty try for Australia soon after, while the Poms had 12 men. But the home side fought back before Wally latched onto a fine offload by hooker Royce Simmons and dummied twice down the short side, then virtually jumped over one defender before splitting the defence and running from the touch line to under the posts to score the try that sealed the match.

His most persuasive try came in the State of Origin match of 1989 at the Sydney Football Stadium, a Queensland victory regarded as their bravest in Origin history. The Maroons had lost Allan Langer (broken leg), Mal Meninga (fractured eye socket), Paul Vautin (elbow) and Michael Hancock (shoulder), leaving them with 13 players and no replacements as the Blues, led by executioner-style prop Peter Kelly, had bashed them (to use a league figurative description). With the crowd deriding him all night, King Wally scored one of Origin's great individual tries by splicing open the defence with a 'show and go', displaying deceptive speed to run 30 metres diagonally to the right and holding off the defence, which anticipated he would stall and look for support, before taking NSW fullback Garry Jack over the line with his brute strength. Queensland, forced to finish the game with 12 men after Bob Lindner could no longer battle on with a fractured ankle, won 16–12.

Soon after, however, the juggernaut started to slow. He was dumped as Brisbane captain in a controversial decision by Wayne Bennett that caused enormous statewide emotional debate, had knee surgery and was then controversially ruled out of the 1990 Kangaroo tour with a broken arm (suffered three months earlier), despite playing a club game, passing a fitness test and being long-time Australian captain. An orthopaedic specialist, Merv

Cross, had been called in to inspect his x-rays and he disagreed with Wally's own surgeon, Dr Peter Myers, by declaring him unfit to tour. Claims of an interstate conspiracy were quickly promoted. In that same year (1990) he had become unwanted by the Broncos and went on to finish his illustrious 14-season career with two seasons finishing last with the Gold Coast Seagulls, his final year in what had become regarded as a redundant role as captain–coach. In the meantime, the day he was due to play for Queensland in the deciding game of the 1991 series, he and wife Jacqui found that their youngest child Jamie-Lee was profoundly deaf, prompting a spontaneous decision to quit representative football that night. In 1993, he left the Seagulls on unhappy terms after one season as non-playing coach, while in 1994 he ended two years as Queensland coach, losing both series 2–1. That snapshot confirms how controversy was his regular partner.

Wally's biography (*King Wally*), written by author Adrian McGregor, was the first of its genre in 1987 (months before the autobiography of New South Wales' similar love him/hate him character Ray Price), and has been updated and re-released three times (1989, 1993, 2004) under varying titles. That is unprecedented for an Australian sporting figure and reflects his standing, particularly in parochial Queensland.

So, his eventful rugby league career I have just prefaced has been endlessly documented. He became a national figure so well recognised, and held in such awe by most Queenslanders almost two decades after his last appearance for the state, that it is almost incomprehensible. However, this is the first time he has opened himself up, first person, in a book. It mostly involves his life post-football and provides an insight into a less public side of Wally Lewis.

What wasn't widely known until the day before his 48th birthday was his suffering of epilepsy that ran parallel with what so many saw as the near-perfect career, just as bipolar disorder was to privately shadow Andrew Johns' great achievements. Wally's vulnerability was exposed ingloriously as he had a seizure while presenting the sports news for Channel 9 in Brisbane, confirming that serious medical conditions do not discriminate.

The Wally Lewis of more recent years was a different character to the one that conquered all before him on the field. The brashness was replaced with an eroding of confidence because of the uncertainty of his epileptic 'auras'; the air of invincibility and cockiness turned to almost a shyness at times; the willingness to be outspoken became less prevalent. His son Mitchell perhaps best described Wally's frustration at watching epilepsy gradually strangle his life's enjoyment with: 'King Wally could always see the opponent; he knew what the opponent was going to do and he knew how to beat it; but this was something completely different.'

Wally now tells this compelling story. He is just one of many epilepsy sufferers and is the kind who does not thrash about on the floor with 'grand mals' but suffers 'auras' where he goes into a brief state of confusion, losing control of speech, thought and sometimes body. His fate should not be, and isn't in this book, over-dramatised as tens of thousands share his affliction and learn to live quite 'normally' with the illness, although many others have had their quality of life severely affected. Wally has met, counselled and supported many of them and considers himself a fortunate one.

What makes his story fascinating, however, is how it affected a very public life and how he tried to live a charade for two decades, hiding it from others as he attempted to palm off its intrusion with medication, until he was cornered into a situation where major surgery was his only saviour. The salvation his operation brought took him to a point where he is comfortable now sharing the story of his private life in the hope it will increase awareness about others like him who suffer epilepsy.

ONE

FLASHPOINT

'Sixty seconds until we're back.'

It was a regular call from the floor manager during the commercial break that led into the Channel 9 Queensland sports bulletin. But it had become more than a standard lead-in for me; it was also the countdown to a time bomb within my body. One that was never planned or scheduled.

And I was thinking, 'Will it go off tonight?'

It was 29 November 2006. Immediately before the commercial break I'd delivered a short description of what was to come in sport before settling back comfortably into the chair. The break gave me a chance to practise my delivery of the upcoming stories, and a short period of ease before the countdown began. It wasn't unusual to feel uncomfortable but the quick self-assessment which had become standard procedure told me I was okay, albeit nervous. Very nervous.

I had already been over the introduction to my opening story five or six times, and had little difficulty. I was breaking out into a light sweat but thought, and hoped, that was probably just due to the heat generated by the powerful lighting setup overhead, standard for every television studio.

It was common for the newsreading team to remain light-hearted while off camera, and the Nine news anchors Bruce Paige and Heather Foord had always been of great assistance that way. Heather and I regularly wished each other 'all the worst' for the upcoming bulletin and with Pagey being a keen footy fan we'd all become pretty close over the years. They'd become invaluable allies, real professionals. But even decades of covering dramatic stories would prove worthless that night when the drama occurred right before their eyes on the newsroom floor.

The half-minute warning certainly increased my heart rate. I could feel the adrenalin racing throughout the veins, as it was something I'd experienced thousands of times before, especially on the football field. But the expectation of springing into action quickly drowned as panic started to set in.

'Twenty seconds …'

After that call pierced the otherwise silent studio, another tingling feeling pumped through my system. It was an indication that I was about to have a 'turn', or 'seizure' as it is known medically. 'No, not now ... not here,' I pleaded with myself.

Apparently I dropped my head in Heather's direction and whispered, 'Oh no.' She was confused by my comment, but there was more of a surprise to come.

'Ten ... nine ... eight ... seven ... six ...'

I tried to quickly race over the script to prepare for the first line.

'Five ... four ... three ... two ... one.' I was on camera. It was the point of no return.

Until then, I could understand what was written on my script, but just as the floor manager silently directed his finger at me to begin delivering the first story, I froze. All the words in front of me were blatantly obvious, but I couldn't comprehend them. Even delivering the first couple of words proved impossible.

Inside the control room, the news director reacted quickly and pushed the 'vision' button, as the story rolled without any introduction. There were plenty of other things missing too; my pride and dignity being among them.

I can remember Heather turning to me to ask if I was okay, but I don't recall if I said anything in reply or, if I did, whether it could have possibly made sense.

But I do remember wondering if I'd done something else to further embarrass myself. Was I dribbling from the mouth? Had I urinated everywhere while I was sitting there?

I hadn't. Thank God. Not like the last time.

That was 13 days earlier when, in almost identical circumstances, I had a seizure just as the camera centred upon me after the commercial break had finished, before which I'd been fine previewing what was to come in sport.

That's about as demeaning and embarrassing as you could get; pissing yourself while sitting in the chair next to two colleagues on the news set. At least that time Bruce was able to take over before I began to deliver the report. This time I wasn't so lucky.

On the first occasion, we'd been able to fob off the media with a story that I'd been ill from a virus, as evidenced by me having recently lost a lot of weight. I knew straight away, second time around, that there was no dodging the truth or dodging any more bullets while on air.

I thought my television career had ended right then and there.

The next sight Queensland Channel 9 viewers saw was Bruce Paige delivering the rest of the sports news. What they couldn't see was me sitting there, frozen; humiliated.

I was in total confusion. I felt I'd insulted the station …
again. And I'd embarrassed myself in front of two million
people, in what I regarded as the lowest point of my life
— well, at that stage.

I declared myself to be okay and remained in the chair
until the end of the bulletin. The seizure had passed and I
walked straight back to the sports room, and my office —
it was the loneliest 30 metres I'd ever paced. By then, there
were plenty of things racing through my mind, interrupted
only by the ring of my mobile phone that sat on my desk.

It was my wife Jacqui, who'd been calling the office
number non-stop since the incident took place. She was
screaming and crying hysterically and struggled to
complete a single sentence. Although I assured her that
everything was fine, she was in an obvious state of panic.
My eldest son Mitchell sat her down and took over the
conversation, arranging to come and collect me.

But there were other things to be picked up. I began
clearing my desk before I was joined by the chief news
editor Ron Kruger. Ron and I had become good friends
over the years and had always enjoyed long conversations
about sport, particularly football and cricket. Ron's son
Nick had excelled, representing Queensland in one-day
and Sheffield Shield cricket. On this occasion we were
initially both lost for words.

Eventually I broke the ice. I couldn't stop apologising for what I'd done to Channel 9's credibility and told him I couldn't put him in that situation again; I was jumping before I was pushed. After the previous episode it was station manager Lee Anderson who was first to greet me in my office and, as politely as he could, he'd told me, 'This can't keep going on ...' I interrupted with, 'Mate, if you want me to pull up stumps, I will. I know I can't keep going on like that.' I interpreted his comment as a warning that my job was in jeopardy, which was totally understandable. However, Lee assured me he was suggesting I just had to come clean that I suffered epilepsy and get something done about my condition, and he was there to support me, which he certainly has done since.

I'd played Russian roulette long enough. It was obvious this time that I couldn't live my life like that any more. I'd already insulted myself, my family and the station enough. I couldn't damage the integrity of Channel 9 any longer. I had to walk. I knew I still owed a huge apology to Lee and my sports boss Andrew Slack, who'd left for a function just before the news bulletin commenced, but that could come later.

Ron kept trying to assure me that my job wasn't the important thing just then, but getting me healthy was. We spoke for about 10 minutes — while the switchboard and my mobile phone were going crazy; the media were wanting to know what was going on, as were viewers. While I greatly appreciated his support and compassion, I didn't think I could ever return. He kept saying, 'Don't worry about it; don't worry about it,' and I said, 'Ron, I can't do this to you again, mate. I have to get rid of this; I have to do something.'

As far as I know, Ron, Lee and 'Slacky' were the only ones at the station who were aware of my condition. In 2002 or 2003, three or four years into my career at Nine, I confided in Slacky after he'd obviously observed one night that there was something wrong with me. He'd looked at me quite concerned and said, 'You alright, mate?'

I'd got into the habit of disappearing out of view when I felt an 'aura' or 'seizure' coming on during the day and heading straight to the toilet until it passed. Finally, I told Slacky that, no, I wasn't alright. I spilled out what was wrong with me and about my one great fear: that I would screw up on air; that I'd have a turn right there in front of the camera.

Well, that time had come — that great fear had just been realised. I'd reached the lowest point.

Another good friend at Nine, Steve 'Spanner' Hopgood, soon arrived in the office and arranged to deliver me to my sons at the arranged collection point a few kilometres from the studios. Ha, wasn't that an ironic location ... Suncorp Stadium.

Rarely did I not enjoy visiting Suncorp, or Lang Park as we knew it in the great old days during my football career. I had virtually grown up at the ground after playing my first game there in 1967 as an eight-year-old. Both sets of grandparents lived within 300 metres of the fences; it was almost my second home, as well as the headquarters of rugby league in Queensland — 'The Cauldron' that had completely mesmerised me as an aspiring young footballer. It had become the scene of some of my proudest moments, but meeting my two sons Mitchell and Lincoln after the events of that night certainly wasn't one of them.

Upon their arrival, my sons didn't have much to say. They were trying to remain calm, but Lincoln didn't hide his concern too well. Mitchell was obviously very concerned but had taken the big brother approach and tried to settle Linc's fears. Any time the three of us got into a car, it was usually a fairly talkative affair, with plenty of laughing and storytelling, but on this occasion the conversation remained brief. Perhaps they were a little confused, but they knew any show of anxiety or panic from them wasn't going to do much good ... there was obviously plenty of that awaiting at home.

Usually my dogs are the first to greet me upon my arrival home after work; but not on this occasion. Plenty of relatives were on hand, and they certainly hadn't come to check on the Christmas gifts or because they happened to be in the neighbourhood. They were there to calm and support Jacqui and be there for me. But I was in no socialising mood. And as hard as it was to politely avoid conversation in my house, there was also the media from Brisbane and Sydney, Gold Coast and Townsville, who'd already clogged up my voicemail with a heap of messages. I didn't answer one of them; I didn't mean to be rude, but I just felt like being alone on the seat in the living room that had become my haven so often when I was feeling down and just wanting a bit of time to myself.

Time on my own was becoming a more regular occurrence. I knew epilepsy had largely taken over my life and had almost turned me into a hermit. Conversation was no longer something I revelled in amongst friends; at times I found it difficult to become involved in widespread discussion. It wasn't something that I'd noticed as much as others did, to be honest. When I was involved in a conversation I'd sometimes pause before completing the sentence. I was later told that the delay sometimes lasted up to five or six seconds. Some attributed it to me simply thinking about another thing that had crossed my mind, while others quietly assumed it may have been long-term damage suffered from playing such a physical contact sport as rugby league.

That night I couldn't even attempt to talk. I didn't want to let those in the house know how I felt and what I might do; and I couldn't have contemplated how I would have explained it if I'd wanted to. I'd just made a complete dickhead of myself in front of two million people and I was absolutely devastated. I sat there forever, it seemed, only getting out of my chair to say goodbye to people — and I don't think I even got up to do that a couple of times.

The rest of that night was tough, and long, as my whole life flashed before me. Even after I went to bed I stared at the ceiling wondering what was going to happen the following day, let alone the rest of my life.

One part of that question was answered pretty early with a knock on the door from the media contingent that had gathered outside. Jacqui deflected them the best she could with the line that we didn't know what my illness was, and until I'd had tests there was nothing to say.

I'd lived with the secret of being an epileptic for over 20 years by then and had confided in very few people; I went to great pains for it to be my battle and not a public one. More people than I'd wanted to found out through the grapevine, but still nothing had come out in the media, even after my on-screen turn the fortnight earlier. This time, though, the news reporters sniffed a story.

Later that day, Jacqui and I went to see Noel Saines, my specialist at the Wesley Hospital, and went through all the normal questions and answers. As I told Noel, what happened had been just the same as the previous one and the many before that, except on this particular occasion I couldn't have picked a worse time or place. He spoke of the options available to help control the seizures and improve my quality of life. I was already on probably the maximum dosage of medication possible — I was taking four different drugs in Tegretol, Dilantin, Topomax and Keppra. He said something like, 'And as we've mentioned before, one option is surgery.' I gulped!

Noel had previously mentioned surgery several times. I remember telling him around the third or fourth visit many years earlier that I'd consider surgery as an option if the medication continued to fail controlling the seizures. But more recently, I'd pushed it out to option 'd', 'e' or 'f'. Later, I pushed it out to option 'z' and even if we reached it then I would have changed it to a numerical option, knowing the path to infinity would take a while. Something happened that assured me there was no way I was going down that path; I'll explain later in the book.

Jacqui was present the first time Noel discussed possible surgery, many years before, but had no idea I'd dismissed it outright at any mention since; I never alerted her that it had even come up in conversation, especially not in my previous visit. When he brought it up in front of her, she glared at me, amazed and angry. 'You've never told me that *that* [surgery] had been mentioned again,' she said with those piercing eyes. As it turned out, the timing of the revelation was ironic because I had reached such a low, I'd put up the white flag. Suddenly the surgery I'd been so pessimistic about looked the only way out.

We'd become good friends with Peter Silburn and his wife Suellen through social and sporting events via our daughters both attending All Hallows School in Brisbane; our Jamie-Lee, who is profoundly deaf, and their daughter Eloise. It wasn't until much later that I found that Peter was, in fact, Professor Peter Silburn, respected surgeon and neurologist and one of Queensland's experts on Parkinson's disease and Tourette's Syndrome.

A couple of days after seeing Noel Saines, Jacqui thought it would be good to confide in Peter. I visited him one evening after he'd finished his duties for the day.

It was more a confession than a discussion; I did all the talking for over an hour and Peter just intercepted with the 'What happened next?', 'How long did that go on for?', 'How did it make you feel?' sort of questions. Towards the end, tears were welling in my eyes and he cut it short with, 'Well, mate, you're going to Melbourne to see Professor Sam Berkovic. There are three men in the world at the top of the tree when it comes to epilepsy, and he's one of them. There are some good people in Brisbane, but if we want the best, he's it.' Thankfully, I took Peter's advice.

In the meantime, the night after crashing so embarrassingly in front of the camera, I let out my secret about epilepsy in an interview with Nine that other news outlets soon took up. The lying, the hiding, the anxiety and the helplessness that I'd been able to keep buried for so long were released. The next day, 1 December, was my 48th birthday … the ordeal wasn't much of a present.

They often say in life you have to reach the bottom to finally work your way out of a hole. That was the case with me. It was a tough, rough, long road after that for a while as I slowly recovered from the major surgery. And if I'd thought the deep disgrace and embarrassment I felt those two nights on the news desk would be the lowest points, soon afterwards I was wrong.

ANOTHER PERSPECTIVE

By Bruce Paige, Channel 9 Brisbane news presenter

16 November 2006, episode 1

It was a normal night. I threw to Wally and he previewed the upcoming sport stories, and we settled down during the commercial break.

Wal seemed a bit agitated. I put that down to him having the flu. He decided to proceed and got out a 'good evening' before his read became unintelligible. The director went straight to the story and I was asked to complete the sport break. Between story 'intros' (and I'm glad I didn't have to name any cricket players from the sub-continent) we were checking on Wally. Almost as quickly as the episode came on, it was over. But I remember thinking how annoyed Wal was with himself. After the bulletin, Wal was very down and taken off to hospital for tests.

29 November 2006, episode 2

When it happened again about a fortnight later, we all began to realise it wasn't just the flu. Again Wally recovered during the sports break, but he really looked as though he wanted to open a vein. Later, walking to the car, I had a call from a sports reporter mate of Wal's asking after his condition, and for the first time the 'E word' was used.

With the benefit of hindsight, I say, 'How tough is this bloke?' Knowing what could happen, he still fronted up each and every night and delivered the sports news. I reckon prepping up for each night's read would have been as taxing as readying himself for a State of Origin game. But then again there are only three of those a year.

ANOTHER PERSPECTIVE

By Heather Foord, Channel 9 Brisbane news presenter

In the weeks before Wally's worst seizure on air, at the end of November 2006, I'd been becoming increasingly concerned about his behaviour. Occasionally he would be extremely vague, and what I took as extremely nervous when about to read the sport during the news half-hour.

Being 'The King', a famous but very private man, nobody really wanted to embarrass him by asking what was wrong. I put it down to nerves, and too many head knocks during his career. So I did what we did best together — I just teased and ribbed him as usual (nicely, of course) — hoping that would relax him.

But that night was different.

Going into the commercial break he seemed fine — relaxed even. But as soon as the countdown ended, he froze, then stammered. I realised he wasn't going to recover. So I signalled to the floor manager to change the shot — fortunately the director had the same idea — and went to the taped story.

But Wally was in dire straits. He was shaking uncontrollably down his right side, and the air was full of the scent of panic. I reached over and held his hand — hard — to try to make him stop shaking, and he still wasn't making any sense.

As we helped him out of the studio, he said, 'Well, that's it then. I don't know when I'll be back — if ever.' I was panicked and worried … but we had to finish the bulletin, so someone else took him to the men's room.

The rest is history.

The thing that bothered me most was that Wally could have endured epilepsy for so long, and so badly, but we, who worked with him every night, had no idea.

His resulting operation was both a brave and dangerous thing to have to choose — but for Wally, there was no choice. He had hit the bottom, privately, and by then publicly, and there was only one alternative to surgery, and that was unthinkable.

I was never a footy fan, so had little idea of his past glories, but I've since learned a lot about Wally and how courageous and inspiring he is. And it's got nothing to do with rugby league.

TWO

THE START

MOST people can remember a significant 'first': their first kiss, first time they got drunk, their first car; yeah, I better add first sexual experience too. I had absolutely no idea what I'd encountered until many years later, but I can certainly remember the first time I had an epileptic seizure.

It was just a normal footy-season Sunday morning. It was the same old routine: I'd have a quiet night and be up for breakfast in time to sit in front of the television by 9am at our family home in Cannon Hill to catch the start of *Sports Scene*, on which a panel would discuss the day's sport, particularly rugby league, for a couple of hours.

It was 1980, I was 20 and in my third season of first grade with the Fortitude Valleys club, playing lock, and was fortunate to be in a successful side. In my first season in 1978 we made the grand final but went down 14–10 to Easts (a loss we avenged the next season by whipping Souths 26–0, who were coached by Wayne Bennett and had Mal Meninga in the centres), and I'd developed a real determination to make some sort of career out of rugby league and to play representative football for Queensland.

It was an important day for me as I'd been selected as lock in the Brisbane 'City' side to play Queensland Country at Lang Park that afternoon and had trained with the Brisbane team all week. There'd been a fair bit of debate surrounding my selection ahead of Brisbane Wests' Norm Carr, who'd held the position for Brisbane and Queensland for five or six years and had been generally regarded for a long time as unquestionably the best lock in the state. I was determined to take full advantage of the opportunity that afternoon, but as it turned out it was a benchmark day for a completely different reason.

I'd settled in to watch *Sports Scene* with my breakfast on my lap and had been there for a while when I felt this flush go through me. I'll describe it as I have plenty of times since to doctors: as funny as it seems, it's kind of like having an orgasm. This tingling goes through your body as if something is building up inside of you and you can't stop it. And that's what happened that morning; something just went through my body and I couldn't control it.

Suddenly I couldn't understand what the panelist was saying. He said something like 'and that's the way it should be this afternoon at Lang Park', and all I could pick up was 'at ... should ... Lang Park ... way... this afternoon ... Lang Park ... should ... that's'. The words seemed to be going backwards, sideways, all out of place; it was completely dyslexic. At the end of that segment it felt like I'd heard it all before, even though I couldn't understand what was being said. It was truly bizarre. I was probably in that state for a minute and a half wondering what the hell was going on with me. I tried to talk but I couldn't; nothing would come out. Then I broke into a cold sweat.

I called out to my mother and both my parents came in. I just sat there shaking my head and tried to explain what had happened and how I was feeling. They decided they'd take me straight to the family doctor at Wynnum, about 12 kilometres away. I shrug when I think of it today; we always seemed to drive out to Wynnum when it would have been far quicker to go into a hospital in the city. I suppose the comfort of having the familiarity of your regular doctor was important and, in those days, a drive to the casualty ward was considered only if you had a threatening injury or illness.

Anyway, I explained to the doctor what had happened and he said, 'Mate, you've got the flu.' He told me there was this particular strain of flu going through the city and my symptoms sounded very much like it was that. He gave me antibiotics and we accepted his diagnosis.

When I got home I still felt terrible and had no choice but to pull out of the match. Norm Carr started as lock and after his usual good performance was picked for Queensland for the first interstate game as captain, and I missed the squad.

I'd also copped a knock to the head against Wynnum Manly the previous weekend and had bad headaches and a bit of dizziness for a couple of days afterwards. So I was sent to the Mater Hospital for some tests next day to be on the safe side, but I was cleared of anything other than a virus.

After missing the first interstate match I was chosen as halfback for the second game against New South Wales. A few weeks later, I was fortunately selected at lock (with Norm Carr a reserve) for the first-ever State of Origin game that followed the two 'regular' interstate matches that New South Wales had won 35–3 and 17–7. Queensland won the historic Origin clash at Lang Park 20–10, so the representative season that began with my withdrawal from the Brisbane side because of a 'flu-type virus' didn't end so badly.

I seemed to cop a dose of the flu pretty badly two or three times a year from then — always in the football season — although I seemed to be able to shake it off and never worried a great deal about it. Like any 19 or 20 year old, I was often going out and getting on the grog and not doing what your mother tells you often enough, like keeping a jumper on when it got cool in the evening or getting a good amount of sleep. I'd get the sniffles or full-blown flu every now and again and just put it down to not looking after myself like my mum said I should have been.

I was always out with my mates and loved a beer. Pretty often, certainly outside of football season, I would have three or four hours' sleep Friday night, then four or five the next night and plenty of beers in between, which would obviously knock me around. Once the surf season started, I'd go down to the Gold Coast just about every weekend with a few mates; most often with the boys who would ultimately be in my bridal party — Brian Ball (best man) and Alan Mohle (groomsman).

We were members of Nobby Beach Surf Club and we'd go down there Friday evenings, arriving about 7pm. About 50 blokes would shack up for two nights, and after we'd claimed our beds we'd retire to the surf club bar for a few beers and a lot of laughs or, often, a lot of beers and a few laughs! We'd stay up until all hours in the morning; there was a rule that there was no sleep for the weekend and you were weak if you called it quits early.

We'd also do our bit with the surf patrol over the weekend and maybe compete in a carnival on the Sunday. Then we'd get home when it was dark and try to catch up on some shut eye that had been sacrificed the previous two nights. By the time I'd reached 21 I was thinking I was too old for that summer lifestyle, when it was obvious it was starting to knock me around too much.

The following year I had the 'turns' a couple of times in two days at one stage and I was a bit worried. I went back to the family surgery and saw a different doctor this time — he told me I just had a bad dose of influenza again. He said it wasn't uncommon that when you get hit by the flu you can get hot and cold sweats and you can feel a surge go through you and feel weak. I had no reason to doubt him, and again, after I took a course of antibiotics I seemed to feel better for the next few months.

From then, I might get the 'feeling' two or three times over a few days and feel clogged up and run down for a while; then I'd be okay for weeks or months. After that season I had a good period with none of the previous sort of episodes for a year or more. When I did get the 'surges', they'd only last 15 to 30 seconds and didn't worry me too much.

Little did I know what they really were.

THREE

THE DIAGNOSIS

MY football, and life generally, were going well: I'd achieved the honour of captaining Queensland and Australia and I married Jacqueline in November 1984. However, after a long period without those nasty bouts of the 'flu', the strange 'surges' started to become more regular in 1986–87, although they seemed to pass without any great drama. I lived with them; I just accepted them as part of life.

I'd never had any major faint-headedness or moments of confusion on the football field; well, none that I could identify as anything other than a bit of concussion from a head knock. Until, that is, the one-off Test match against New Zealand at Lang Park on 21 July 1987. It was played just six days after Queensland had beaten New South Wales 10–8 in a really physical deciding Origin match, also at Lang Park, in which I copped a black eye and sore 'melon'.

That Test match became a night I'd rather forget for a few reasons. Firstly, after going through the 1986 Kangaroo tour undefeated for a second occasion and Australia winning all nine Tests the previous season, we got touched up 13–6 by an inexperienced Kiwi team that fielded quite a few players who were regarded as 'no names' at that time. Secondly, my head came off second best in a collision with their fullback Darrell Williams' knee, after I went to tackle him head on. My head went right forward, my chin hit my chest; I heard a crack and pain shot down my neck. It's not a nice feeling and you naturally fear the worst in that moment when you hear that sound and you've got pins and needles down your arms. I stayed down until I could get the right attention, but I came good and was able to get up and play out the match.

That night was also significant as it was the first time I had what I now realise was a seizure on the football field. It came well before the ill-fated tackle on Darrell Williams. I'd gone into another tackle and had made the cardinal mistake of not placing my head in the correct position when effecting a tackle. From your first training session as a young boy, you're taught to place your head to the side of a player running directly at you and make contact with your shoulder; or, if you're making a side-on tackle, to place your head behind the man. That ensures you won't be hit by the ball carrier's knees during his sprint or have the attacking player fall on you. No matter how many times it was preached and practised, I still made the occasional mistake. And when I did, I never forgot the consequences. I still recall *that* feeling clearly. Describing it is somewhat difficult, but it always reminded me of the introduction to a Rank movie, where a man standing alongside a massive drum would strike it with a large lump of wood. *Gonnnggg!!*

When you attempt to get to your feet quickly, your disorientation is obvious. Your balance is completely gone and your body keeps falling in one direction, but the more you attempt to regain balance by leaning the other way, the worse it seems to become. It's followed by a feeling of, 'Oh no, I've done it again — I'm back in Disneyland,' and a massive loss of confidence hits you as you try to battle on, knowing you're still hazy.

But this one was a little different in that sounds became inaudible around me and there was more confusion than usual; and while I felt faint, I didn't feel groggy. I put it down to concussion, just a bit different to what I'd had many times before. But now that the feeling I had that night is far more common to me, I can identify it as an epileptic seizure. It was very disturbing.

Losing the game was another thing that left me feeling uncomfortable that night. My mood immediately after a defeat wasn't something that promoted good sportsmanship. Jacqueline is an effervescent character who doesn't mind a bit of a chat, but she quickly learned that talking to me after a loss was simply a one-way conversation; like talking to a post. And if that loss occurred in a Test or State of Origin match, my mood would be even filthier. For hours, I'd replay the game in my mind, attempting to discover the reasons behind the disaster. The old saying, 'It doesn't matter whether you win or lose, it's how you play the game,' is very important in the promotion of sport for kids. But my response to any advocate of that notion at senior level was: 'Bullshit. If that's the case, I'm glad you're not in my team.'

So I was feeling bloody rotten after losing that Test match, and the fact I had a sore head, crook neck, crook knee and a dose of concussion didn't help my mood. After I'd cooled down, the ARL doctor, Dr Kevin Hobbs, checked me out and decided to put me in a neck brace as a precaution. While talking to him I mentioned that I also had this funny feeling during the game, and described it to him. Considering I'd copped a bad head knock and was momentarily unconscious in the Williams tackle, he seemed quite concerned. 'That doesn't sound good; we better get you straight into the Wesley Hospital and check you out.' So I was taken out of Lang Park on a stretcher, put into an ambulance and escorted to hospital.

The following morning, doctors spent a lengthy period questioning me. They seemed to go away for a while only to come back with another query, then another. The points discussed included the frequency of my 'turns', the levels of confusion when they occurred, and whether there was any family history of serious medical disorders. The only one I knew of was my mother's coronary complaints, as she had struggled with palpitations of the heart and had spent time in hospital because of them. But there seemed to be an eye or two raised when I mentioned the frequency with which I seemed to be troubled by the 'flu' and just how confused I became during these 'short spells'. When I mentioned the strange feelings that passed through me, I was referred to a specialist.

I had all the regulation x-rays and scans, but I'd had a few overnighters in hospital before and wasn't too worried. The tests cleared me of any serious neck damage; I'd suffered strained ligaments and also torn cartilage tissue in my knee. But the doctor told me they wanted to conduct more tests on my brain.

Soon after a doctor came in and introduced himself as Dr Douglas Killer. I didn't know if he was serious or not; at first I thought he was geeing me up and I said something like, 'Yeah sure, good one.' But when I looked at his hospital identification I nearly slumped to the floor in embarrassment. I apologised but Douglas replied, 'Don't worry, I cop that all the time.'

Anyway, Doug, who was in charge of the neurological ward, quickly got down to business and said he wanted to carry out another test 'just to clear a few things up'. I was transferred to the radiology department for some more scans, a place that has since become very familiar territory. I'd been there before, following concussions, but this was to be a little different and the visit lasted a lot longer than usual. Meanwhile, I'd been told that a rather large media contingent was outside awaiting my discharge. Thankfully Jacqueline had brought in a change of clothes. Facing the cameras in either the smelly Australian jersey you'd played a full match in, or the Australian blazer you'd worn to the game, would ensure a lengthy bagging from your team-mates, who'd accuse you of being a lair.

I still didn't suspect there was anything wrong with me, so I asked if I could shower and get ready to be discharged. A nurse advised me that Douglas was coming back to see me and Jacqui and I had to wait. It turned out to be an appointment that changed my life.

Entering the room with a smile is probably standard procedure for doctors, and when he walked in I was expecting a 'you're clear to go' instruction, such was the look upon his face. But when he asked me to sit down for a while, I knew there was something else coming. He introduced the news by telling me all the tests had been done and there were no apparent problems from the concussion. However, his next question left me stumped: 'Does anyone in your family suffer from epilepsy?' After I replied that there was no known history of it, he slowly advised me that more tests may have to be done, but the scans indicated that I did … suffer … epilepsy. I was an *epileptic*!

'No, not me; that can't be right,' I demanded. 'There's no history of it in the family anywhere.' Jacqui squeezed my hand tightly. I wanted another series of tests conducted; I wanted to check whether it was right or not. I was in complete denial. I'd never had any behaviour that I associated with epilepsy; I'd certainly never had any violent fits.

But the more Douglas discussed the symptoms and the condition, I knew the tests must have been correct. Once again donning the hospital gown, I sat back in my bed, and while I had several hours until the next set of tests was carried out, there was little comfort. Not for me, nor Jacqui, nor for the awaiting journos who were starting to become intrigued by my second day in hospital. And it didn't take long for the rumours to begin; from me bleeding on the brain, to concussion, to a serious neck injury and partial paralysis. Any of these scenarios would have made a good story.

In all, I spent three days having tests and receiving advice on how my future should be planned. The advice was to be closely adhered to, I was told; well, warned pretty sternly really. But there was one 'rule' that raised the eyebrows more than any other: no alcohol while you're taking the prescribed medication, Tegretol. Whoa! You can't do that. What am I gonna do with the boys? No beers with the team on a Sunday night after the game? On top of that, I was involved in television commercials for a beer company and was expected to drink at their promotions.

Upon my release, it was time to finally face the waiting media. We were worried about it being a bit of a bun fight and someone suggested I plan an escape via an entry the media wouldn't know of. That would have been foolish — I had to face the media at some stage, and if they missed me at the hospital they would have camped outside our house, so I suggested we just make an announcement at the hospital.

Before I faced the cameras I'd rehearsed how I'd focus my explanation on my neck troubles, declaring that the three-day period was routine when dealing with possible spinal cases. The truth was that my neck was still very uncomfortable and I was wearing a brace around it to reduce discomfort, but I'd been cleared of any serious damage. After declaring that 'the loss to the Kiwis was the most painful thing of all', I relayed that I was no longer under the magnifying glass. It grabbed the headlines and satisfied the media and the public. Little did they know the real story; the real dilemma facing me. Thankfully, nothing ever got out, so the confidentiality of the hospital staff passed the test.

I went home and considered my new challenge. My first reaction was shock. Did I feel any shame or embarrassment? I don't think I felt shame but I certainly didn't want my condition to become public knowledge. Plus, at that stage there was a bit of dissatisfaction with the media on my part — a mistrust of some of them, perhaps — and a bit of a barrier had developed between us. I was worried that if the news got out, it would be around the league world in 24 hours and be quite exaggerated in how it was portrayed. I didn't want all that crap; certainly not the attention. I could see the stories saying I might have a fit on the field, my career was threatened, and all of those sorts of things.

The hardest part was that I had something that I knew absolutely nothing about. Like 95 per cent of the population, I thought if you had epilepsy it meant you took big fits and would be kicking and wriggling everywhere on the floor; that anyone who tried to help you would get an accidental punch in the mouth or kick in the teeth, plus someone would grab your tongue so you couldn't swallow it. I'd never had any of those, so how could I be an epileptic?

I was told you don't have to have the tonic-clonic seizures (formerly known as grand mal seizures); you can have the less intense petit mal seizures (now known as absence seizures) which cause more of a disorientation feeling than an actual 'fit'. In fact, much, much later I found out there were 57 kinds of epilepsy. Half of the confusion was that I didn't know a damn thing about it; the other half was how the hell did I get it?

On that last day at the Wesley, another doctor accompanied Dr Killer to my bed and she asked if I'd ever been badly concussed playing football. Of course I had.

'Would it be three times … four, five?' she asked.

'What, per season, you mean?'

'No, in your life.'

I explained that it would have had to have been at least three or four times a season for 10, maybe 15 years; so a total of 40 to 50. She looked at Douglas in absolute amazement. Obviously when I was playing under-age football in my teens they weren't concussions to the level I copped later on, but they were indeed concussions.

I then had to describe in some detail the degree of the head knocks and the resulting grogginess and treatment; from times when I saw stars in my eyes for two or three minutes to the one when I got knocked rotten and I was pretty crook for quite some time. While it can only rarely be discovered what causes epilepsy in each individual, head injury is a very common cause in young adults and that may have been the case for me. But I was told I could well have just been one of the unlucky ones who discover they develop epilepsy for no apparent reason.

It's also regarded as being highly hereditary; thus all the questions they'd fired at me about family history. Mum and Dad confirmed there were no known cases of epilepsy in either family, so it seemed most likely that a series of head knocks had brought it on. However, much later, things that Mum would say got me to thinking that maybe she had some degree of epilepsy, but never knew about it. She'd tell Jacqui, 'I bet you he feels like this when that happens,' as if she had some inkling what I was going through. Mum did have some 'turns' from when I was a teenager, that became worse as she got older which doctors put down to a heart problem.

I remember when I'd just turned 18 and she made an uncomplimentary comment about my girlfriend of the time. I gave her a real gob-full and walked out of the room.

Next thing, I heard my sister Jeannie screaming that Mum had collapsed on the lounge-room floor. When Mum got up, she kept saying she was alright but I threw her in the car and took her down to our local doctor in Wynnum. Mum had played netball for Queensland and was still playing socially, and she loved playing golf and tennis with her friends. Because she was still very active for her age, it was a bit of a shock for her to go down like that. She was diagnosed as suffering palpitations of the heart and it was attributed to being under pressure — she certainly had turns when she was anxious or stressed.

While it frustrated me to an extent not knowing whether my mother ever had some degree of epilepsy, it didn't surprise me, because that was what it was like in those days. If you were crook and got over it you didn't tell anyone; you didn't broadcast that you were having any difficulties. Whether she was having similar turns to me, we'll never know.

Upon my return home, I had to ensure that there was almost a total change in the lifestyle I'd enjoyed for the previous decade or so. Remembering to take my prescribed medication became something of a daily challenge, and so was dealing with a possible end to my football career. I'd already questioned the doctors about whether a serious head knock had triggered my first 'turn', and I was concerned with the possible dangers if I continued to play. In reality, I knew I didn't want to retire. There were so many things I still wanted to achieve in the game, but I did have a family to look after. Mitchell was just over 12 months old, and Jacqui was heavily pregnant with our second son Lincoln. If it came down to a decision there and then, I would have been like every other proud parent; the kids would have priority.

Thankfully, my introduction to the medication did the trick and the seizures seemed to disappear. There was also a mid-season holiday! With the State of Origin series by then regarded as a showpiece event, just a couple of weeks after the Test match against the Kiwis the Australian Rugby League decided it was time to venture to the United States to promote the code. It was a game players all across the country strived to take part in, although it wasn't the best timing for me in adapting to taking my medication and ensuring ample periods of rest.

Both teams were separated on the Qantas flight to Los Angeles, with New South Wales in the section immediately behind business class, while Queenslanders were at the back of the plane. I'd stayed away from drinking for a couple of weeks but that was to change on that particular trans-Pacific flight. I was seated alongside Queensland front-rower Greg Dowling, and following the mid-flight meal, he ordered a couple of drinks. While I understood that drinking while on medication wasn't advisable, I thought one or two wouldn't hurt. Unfortunately, that led to plenty more. By the time we arrived in Honolulu we were legless, and after reboarding for the flight to LA we tucked into it again.

After a day or two in LA, the penny dropped quite dramatically that drinking was indeed not advisable — I had two episodes in the space of an hour. It was the first time they had been so close.

Following our return to Australia, I ensured there was plenty of rest and relaxation between football games. When I'd arrive home after training sessions Jacqueline would have a hot bath waiting; what a way to relax. The bath was enriching and so were the TV programs I loved watching, like *Fawlty Towers* and *Mother and Son*. But back at my club Wynnum Manly, things weren't quite so comfortable, and the club was announced as being bankrupt soon after. The players hadn't been paid for years. So all in all, I had plenty to contend with in 1987.

Lincoln was born soon after, making 24 October another day I had to have a drink. However, that all changed upon his arrival home, and the two boys booked any spare time I had on the lounge-room floor. Those days playing with them were among the best times of my whole life.

The summer of 1987–88 had me travelling to the doctors on several occasions. I'd had quite a few seizures; sometimes they'd occur immediately after I woke up, other times while I was casually watching television or even mowing the lawn. As requested, I was very careful to record every time they happened and their duration and 'strength'. I recorded the episodes as either light, moderate or heavy. A light turn would usually leave me unable to understand anything that was going on for about 30 to 45 seconds. Medium was around a minute to 90 seconds, while heavy was anything beyond that. I kept those detailed diaries for many years, but I have to admit, my ability to judge the periods was probably not accurate at all. A typical entry would be: 'A turn while watching television. Medium strength. 45–60 secs. Took some time to regain confidence.'

Upon consulting Dr Killer the next time I visited the Wesley Hospital, my medication was once again increased from the initial half a 25 milligram tablet twice a day to taking a full tablet in the morning with another at night. Early the following year that was increased to one-and-a-half tablets morning and night, and I blamed the heavy change in lifestyle, from being part of the Brisbane Broncos during their first season, for my condition deteriorating. The Broncos had been formed to enter the 1988 season against the New South Wales clubs and training at the Broncos was a far busier, and more exhausting, experience than I'd become accustomed to in Brisbane club football.

I was working until 5.15pm at Channel 10 at the time and found myself racing to get to our field at Red Hill in time for the beginning of the session. Once the season began, the matches made the schedule even tougher. On top of training we'd fly to Sydney on average every second week, normally the day before the game, and then have more meetings than the AJC Spring Carnival every time we were away. There'd be one once we'd arrived, another after dinner the evening before the match, then another the following day as the preparation picked up just before we left for the game. After the match had finished there were press conferences to be attended before it was 'busso' back to the airport. After arriving home in Brisbane around 8.30pm, it was off to the Broncos Leagues Club to meet the awaiting supporters. After a couple of hours together there we'd head for home.

During my first year at the club, the turns became much more regular, but it was in my second year that there was a marked increase. I'd have them probably every fortnight — on one occasion during a match — and I'd become very guarded about my condition being 'exposed'. I told as few people as I needed to — I wanted to keep it a secret. And, generally, I was able to do that for the next 20 years.

FOUR

THE SECRET

I REGARDED my epilepsy as a private matter, and I tried hard to keep it that way. When I found I suffered the condition I was captain of the Australian rugby league team and had been diagnosed after being KO'd in a Test match against New Zealand, so I knew what a media story it would be and how it might have been blown up greater than it really was.

Naturally I told my parents, and Jacqui told hers, but beyond them we advised no one initially. And that included my brothers Ed, Scott and Heath and my sister Jeannie, although I'd be surprised if my mother didn't tell them pretty quickly. My old man is the sort of bloke who wouldn't have breathed a word to a soul. Even as my own children grew older over the years, I never mentioned it to them; however, again, I know Jacqui let them know when she thought the time was right.

For many years there were only three people outside of the family that I opened up to. And as far as my memory can fathom, it was early in the 1988 season when I told my best footballing mates, Gene Miles and Paul 'Fatty' Vautin, and my coach at the Broncos, Wayne Bennett.

Despite being on the medication, I'd had a couple of unexpected seizures, and I thought I'd better confide in a couple of my closest friends in case they were around when I had an 'episode'. And while it was probably a safe thing to do, it was something I was to regret later.

Secretly living with epilepsy had been eating away at me for a while. My confidence had received a battering and I suppose I just wanted to explain it to someone. The first person I turned to was 'Geno'. He knew little about epilepsy and was obviously quite shocked; again because my situation didn't involve me having any big fits and thrashing around on the floor. His biggest concern was that I'd had too many head knocks and concussion and that it might be an ongoing problem, especially if I continued to play rugby league.

About the same time I told Fatty. Even though he was in Sydney playing with Manly and I was in Brisbane, we'd remained great mates since playing in under-18 rep teams together, and we'd be on the phone every two or three days bagging the hell out of each other. There was a fair bit of trust between us, so I had no qualms in confiding in Fatty. Like Gene, he was quite shocked and knew little about the varying degrees of epilepsy, but he was very supportive.

The one other person I'd confided in, albeit sometime later, was Wayne Bennett. Although he was my club coach, we were hardly the closest of friends; maybe because we were such different people from different walks of life. However, we had become very close in different areas: one, in our determination to succeed; the other, on the issue of health, seeing as Wayne's son Justin also suffered from epilepsy, and on a couple of occasions had a grand mal seizure whilst attending Saturday morning training sessions. I thought if I told Wayne about my epilepsy he'd understand me a little better and might even give me some guidance on how to cope with it. Perhaps I was also seeking his help, understanding and his support — I'm not sure, but it seemed to be the right thing to do. While it took a while to get it off my chest, I finally informed him, knowing he was one person who would keep it confidential. Typical of Wayne, he never really said much — then or later. But I still felt better that he knew.

There used to be a saying among footballers — most of whom loved to hear and tell any gossip going around the sport — that if you wanted to get an announcement out, you could always rely on the three major communications in the world: telephone, telegram and 'tell a team-mate'. I learned first-hand that that rang true.

It was a few months later, I'd guess during the 1989 season, when we were having a few beers after a match one night at the Broncos Leagues Club and taking the piss out of each other, when my team-mate Allan 'Alfie' Langer said something to me like, 'How you going, Mickey?' The term 'Mickey' had become common to us in relation to a good mate John Crane who suffered from epilepsy; having a mickey was used to describe when he was having a fit.

It seemed to go over the heads of the others within earshot, but not me. I was fuming. I thought, 'How the hell did Alf know?' So I confronted Gene and he stuttered and admitted he'd told Alf I was an epileptic and what to do if I had a fit, explaining that he thought it was best he knew, in case I had a seizure while Gene wasn't around.

I told Gene I was filthy on him and that when I'd confided in him with something so personal, and something he knew I was so determined to keep private, I expected he would honour my request.

The trouble was that when we were all full of grog, there was no doubt someone was liable to let something out without realising. And while I knew Alf was just teasing me there was some concern that someone else may pick it up. And to be honest, Gene and I were probably to blame for some of that. When Alf came into the Queensland State of Origin team as a jockey-sized 21-year-old in 1987, Gene and I targeted him on the drink, and made a mess of him one night by encouraging him to meet our pace with some drinks that were being served in vase-like glasses. The next morning we had to travel to Sydney to prepare for the game, and Alf couldn't rise out of his bed. He may have eventually put on his pants by himself before collapsing back onto the mattress, but our manager Dick 'Tosser' Turner and the other managers had to finish dressing him. And it brought the house down when, after they'd come downstairs, we saw Tosser holding Alf's head up by the chin to keep him still in front of a mirror as he combed Alf's hair, while the little fella looked like he was in a coma. In those days, it took very little for Alf to get drunk.

One night, John Crane and I were both in a small group of people and Alf said something like, 'We've got two Mickeys here tonight.' 'Craney' looked around all surprised and said, 'Well who's the other one?' I just glared at Alf, but he let out that cheeky little laugh and didn't say anything more. Nothing further was said but only Craney and I were in the immediate vicinity, so John would have gathered what Alf was talking about. I reckon

Craney would have questioned him afterwards anyway and Alf would have given me up. I'd never thought of telling John; it was more a case of me listening to what he said the rare times his epilepsy was mentioned and taking in all I could. As strange as it sounds, I was a bit relieved that Craney had some bad turns, in that it made me feel as though I wasn't a one-man show; like a freak that should be in the circus.

I'd known John for quite some time; I first met him when he was working for National Panasonic in Brisbane. When Brisbane won the Panasonic Cup in 1984, I won an award — $20,000 worth of Panasonic gear — and I had to go to the factory and pick out what I wanted; it was Craney who walked me through the showroom. Later, he went to Power's Brewery — the Broncos' first major sponsor — and after that became the Broncos' marketing manager. Eventually I confided in him, because I gathered he'd worked out how to live with epilepsy. I asked him what it was like when he had seizures, which could be pretty big ones, and he remarked, 'Mate, if I ever wake up halfway through having one, I'll tell you,' and started laughing. Good point.

I'm sure Alf mentioned our epilepsy to very few, if anyone, when he was sober, but on the grog the Mickey line would come out when we were together. Seeing as

99 out of 100 blokes wouldn't have had any idea what he was talking about, I was probably a bit more paranoid than I needed to be.

Having said that, I was aware that another of our team-mates, Greg Dowling, also found out before I left the Broncos at the end of the 1990 season. 'GD' asked me something about what it was like when I had fits, and he wouldn't have got his information out of a lolly shop. Even though there was the benefit that if I did have a seizure in front of some of the blokes, they'd be able to provide the right information to the medicos, I still didn't feel comfortable about the way it was slipping out — and to this day I don't know how far the 'secret' spread. I'm pretty sure that, for a long while, it was only those footballers who I was closest to.

I'm obviously never going to be sure of how long Fatty kept my epilepsy entirely to himself. I think it would have been until I finished playing footy in 1992, but I do know that he told Peter Sterling, probably in the mid-1990s when they worked together at Channel 9. Until I told my Channel 9 sports director Andrew Slack in about 2002, I hadn't broken my silence to another soul, other than a very close mate Peter O'Callaghan and, many years later, a television colleague, David Fordham; to be honest I trusted the two more than anyone else.

With that secrecy, though, there was a downside. When my behaviour became a little unusual, it left people guessing what was wrong with me and they were getting no explanations, certainly not from me.

I probably had a few minor seizures on the playing field in my last five seasons, between 1988 and 1992, without really noticing, as they came and passed pretty quickly. But I do remember two that rattled me quite a bit. One occurred while I was playing for the Broncos in 1989 at Lang Park and it was an eerie experience. Play was right up one end of the field and I copped a heavy tackle and felt a bit groggy, like I was concussed. But as I tried to get up, I felt a seizure grip me. Suddenly I could hear the noise of the crowd become warped, like I had glasses — the drinking kind — covering my ears, or had my ear up to a sea shell; real muffled sounds that would fade in and out. Amidst all this confusion and inconsistent sounds, I sort of heard someone say, 'C'mon, get back into the play, Wally.' Well, I thought I heard it, or was I imagining it? The words from the crowd seemed to be going forwards and backwards and sideways and I couldn't make sense of anything. It was bizarre.

Naturally I was concerned about what was wrong with me, but when the trainer came on the field I sort of shook him off and said I was okay; he would have just thought I'd received a bit of a knock and was a bit dizzy for a few moments. My biggest fear was that I was going to stuff up on the field; make a massive error that might cost the match if I couldn't get myself right again. It took me the whole five tackles to get back onside up the other end of the field. I'm sure the crowd thought it was just old Wally malingering again and trying to save energy from his old legs, but it definitely wasn't. Eventually I found my senses and played on, although I didn't feel entirely right for the rest of the match.

From that day I was petrified I'd have a seizure during a game and, not knowing how to deal with it in the heat of battle, let the team down. When I went to the doctor for a check-up a month or two later, I told him I'd had a seizure on the field and he asked me all the circumstances. When I told him I seemed to be getting the turns more regularly, he upped my medication.

But as the drugs I was prescribed seemed to have a lessening effect, I started to stumble a bit with my football capabilities and with my conversation as well. My words would become a little slow and slurred sometimes, or it would take me quite a few seconds to respond to a question, because I'd either be having a seizure and couldn't comprehend what was being said or was coming off an 'aura' that may have happened a little earlier. Only after I came clean with my admission about epilepsy did people confide in me that, when my behaviour was like that, they thought I was drunk or had had too many hits on the head playing football.

Bit by bit, I became less comfortable in group conversations and less confident generally in public as the frequency of the seizures increased. But I still didn't want anyone to know other than those who absolutely needed to.

The hint that my seizures could be brought on by head knocks, or at least heavy collisions in tackles, certainly came home to roost one afternoon at Lang Park — ironically in my last-ever game at the ground I most enjoyed playing at. It was 1992, in my final season of playing with the Gold Coast. That was my second year 'down the road' and I'd taken on the captain–coach position, which had become rare in rugby league.

Just after half-time, I copped a blatant blow to the head in a tackle and was seeing stars; it was all my fault as I'd placed my head in the wrong position whilst attempting a tackle. It would have been close to the worst head knock I had during my career; my head went back and crashed into the ground as I fell to the turf, rendering me unconscious. I was in 'ga ga land' as the trainer came on and steered me to the sideline. Again I started to feel disorientated but at first I wasn't sure if it was a dose of concussion or another seizure, until …

All of a sudden, as the trainer looked down at my shorts, I saw the panic in his eyes as he moved closer to me to sort of shield me from the crowd's view. My eyes followed his and I realised I was pissing myself; there was this stain right through my white shorts. How embarrassing. Pissing myself became a common occurrence when I had seizures and couldn't get myself to the toilet in time. So here was my farewell to Lang Park where I'd had my greatest memories and I was a dribbling, pissing mess. I ended up going back on late in the game, just in time to see Allan Langer break an 18-all deadlock and score the winning try for the Broncos under the posts.

I always used to think my 'turns' settled down after a footy season, as my schedule got less hectic. When I was still playing at the Gold Coast in 1991 and '92 I'd get up early in the morning to work at SeaFM, head home for a while, then go to a weights session before heading to training. We had to travel away for games every second weekend and that really took it out of me, especially when there was an add-on trip from Sydney.

My last two years at the Gold Coast were the worst with the frequency and strength of my seizures. There was one particular occasion that certainly stands out. It was in 1993

— I was coaching only after retiring as a player at the end of the previous season, and also working on the breakfast radio show, reading the sports news. I'd start at the radio station at 6am, so I'd have to be up about 4.45am. If we had an away game interstate, we wouldn't get back until late the Sunday night, and by the time we had a few drinks and mixed with the fans and sponsors, I wouldn't get to bed until well after midnight. Getting good sleep is very important for people who suffer epilepsy, so that lifestyle probably increased my chances of having seizures; although countering that was the great natural lifestyle of living on the Gold Coast.

Anyway, my routine was to work at SeaFM until about 10, then I might go to the gym at Southport or come home, play with one or both of the boys for a while (Mitchell and Lincoln began school while we were on the Coast and Jamie-Lee went to kindergarten), and I might have a nap or just relax and watch TV for a few hours before going to training in the afternoon.

This one day, during school holidays, Jacqui went shopping and took the kids and left me at home by myself. Suddenly, on it came, the worst seizure I experienced. I can't say how long it lasted because I became so disorientated and helpless I just lay on the floor, not able to — or wanting to — get up because I knew I'd fall straight over. It lasted at least half an hour and perhaps well over an hour; it was the one time I definitely had a grand mal, as far as I can work out.

Jacqui came home, walked into the lounge room and could tell I was having a bad seizure. When she witnessed one, she'd panic a bit and fire all these questions at me … but usually I just couldn't take in what she was saying and, even if I could, I couldn't respond. The words just wouldn't come out; and if they could it would have been gobbledy-gook anyway. It used to give me the shits, to be honest; she'd be firing away sentences at me at machine-gun speed but she might as well have been talking to the wall behind me. I used to walk away.

That was the case this time. I got frustrated with the interrogation, and after getting to my feet, I kept walking from room to room to escape her and eventually went into our bedroom and tried to lie down. For some reason I kept getting up and going out the door, then returning again. All of a sudden I heard this screaming and Jacqui was yelling at me, just giving it to me, and looking really distressed. I had no idea that I was standing there pissing all over the bed and on the floor. I had no control over my body. I must have got the old fella out, knowing I had to have a leak and probably thinking I was in the toilet; I really can't explain it.

It must have been a terrible bloody shock for her, and naturally once I came to my senses and realised what had happened, it was very demeaning for me too — wetting yourself like a baby missing his nappy, in front of your wife, is not a good experience. But I used to wet myself regularly; then go and clean my clothes or the sheets or blankets or whatever was affected, and act as if nothing had happened, to save the embarrassment. There was another time during that period on the Gold Coast when I had a seizure and was 'gone' for close to an hour, which I recorded in my diary. I assume this was a 'grand mal'.

It was certainly a tough time for Jacqui. Mitchell had just started school and we'd only recently found out Jamie-Lee was deaf; Jacqui was going to and from Brisbane three or four times a week with her tests and treatment. One afternoon she almost fell asleep and veered off the road, with Jamie-Lee in the car. When she got home she looked at me helplessly and said, 'We have to get back to Brisbane; I can't do this any more.'

Even though we loved living on the Gold Coast, due to my impending split with the Seagulls that ended up being an easy decision to make. So we went home and rented a house at Birkdale, on the bay in Brisbane's south, before we eventually built a house in the suburb and have been living happily there ever since.

As well as my SeaFM experience, I'd also worked with Channel 10 during my playing days at the Broncos, doing sports reporting and reading the sports news some nights. I was keen to remain in the media and began working with Channel 7 in the sports department when we returned to Brisbane, and from 1997 also did weekend match commentary for Fox Sports. So I was in, and around, the media quite a lot. But I'll never know how many people were aware of my battle with epilepsy and to what degree I struggled with it, or whether they second guessed that was the case, because only once did a reporter confront me over rumoured 'health issues'.

It was the Sydney *Daily Telegraph*'s Paul Kent, in either 2001 or 2002, at Davies Park in Brisbane where the New South Wales State of Origin team was training. I was there to do interviews for Channel 7 and was talking to good mate and Fox Sports colleague John McCoy, while Kent was a few feet away talking to other journos. I overheard something like 'If he doesn't have one here' or 'You never know, he might gain some attention by having one here'. I turned around and looked over sheepishly, and a little while later Paul Kent came over to us and said he'd heard plenty of rumours about my health and what could I say about it. I tried to laugh it off and offered a lighthearted insult in return, which 'Macca' laughed at. Then I continued: 'Which rumour do I have to deny this time; it's either I'm taking over a coaching job somewhere or something else, and now it's my health — geez, the rumours never end,' and walked away.

Fortunately Kent never pursued it further and never came out with any suggestion that I had 'health problems'. I'm not sure what he'd heard or from whom, and if he said to me he'd been told I had epilepsy I probably would have denied it anyway. If our conversation was in 2002 (I'm only guessing the date), I assume he probably heard rumours after my meltdown during the recording of *This Is Your Life*. That was the first time I got caught out in front of the camera; the vulnerable and embarrassing moment that I'd feared for so long. And that really rocked me.

Being in the public eye, and with rugby league having such a high profile in New South Wales and Queensland, despite the pains I went to in order to keep my condition private, I suppose it's quite remarkable my condition never came out. I know how persistent the media can be to get their story and I'd had my share of being tracked down when I thought I was out of contact — the most harrowing being after Jacqui, the kids and I went to the west coast of America to escape for a while after I lost the Broncos captaincy in late 1989.

The decision by Wayne Bennett hadn't been made public before we left, but it was obviously let out while we were kicking back and showing Mitchell and Lincoln Disneyland and other sights. We pulled into a motel between San Francisco and Los Angeles one afternoon and when the phone in the room rang, I thought, 'Who the hell could that be, no one knows we're here.' It was Peter Kelly, a reporter from Channel 10 where I worked, asking if he could arrange an interview about me being sacked as captain — he told me that the station's US-based journalist had a helicopter ready to come down with a crew. It was just incredible — how could they have tracked me down where I was staying, when we hadn't even made a booking at the hotel?

The next day we pulled into a motel in San Francisco and a heap of messages from media outlets were waiting for me. We had pre-booked that motel, but I still racked my brain over how the hell they could have found us on the other side of the world. I can only assume they either rang a heap of motels at random until they came across my booking, or maybe they had access to a search on my credit card.

With regard to keeping my epilepsy away from public attention, the things that worried me most about my diminishing ability to contain my seizures were lack of sleep, too much alcohol or having an episode live on camera. Although I was doing promotions for Power's during my time playing with the Broncos and then for Carlton and United in ensuing years, I curbed my alcohol intake quite a bit. My work involved plenty of lunches where the host's brew was in ample supply, but I got around that by sipping very slowly, always drinking light beer and having a three-quarters-full glass in my hand most of the time. I remember a couple of occasions when I was doing promos for Carlton and I'd fill a stubby up with ginger beer so it looked like I was drinking the right product. As far as I was concerned, it was about promoting it, not me drinking it.

I used to do a lot of guest speaking but I shied away from that a bit because I was worried that, during the half an hour to an hour I'd be up talking and being interviewed, I was very exposed if a seizure came on. But I worked out a strategy to cover that — I had someone put together a highlights video package from my playing career and, when I needed a break, I'd introduce the video and whack it on. Prior to every guest speaking event, I would create a 'safety net' for myself after being introduced to the crowd.

I'd thank them for their welcome and then say, 'Look, I've been a bit crook lately and I am an asthmatic (which I am), so if I do struggle at any stage I'll just whack on a video of my career highlights and if I'm still crook at the end of that, I'll ask somebody else to come up and finish it off for me. So if there's some poor bastard out there that isn't real good looking and has a hair loss problem, you're in.' Usually it would draw a laugh and tended to add a little relief to the upcoming presentation. Two or three times I felt a turn coming and I'd quickly excuse myself, and by the time the video had finished, the seizure had passed.

I'd make sure I got plenty of sleep during the nights leading up to a speaking gig and would often try to grab an hour's nap, if I could, before I went to the function. I didn't really know if it helped or not, and whether it made me feel more tired or fresher, but I figured I was restocking the supplies of energy and that would give me a better chance of avoiding a seizure.

Having conversations, particularly in groups, was stressful at times. I would look around at the company, check who I was in front of and how well I knew them. If I didn't feel confident, I'd worry that something might go wrong and I'd have a seizure; it increased the fear factor.

Quite honestly, I preferred to stay home whenever I could and if I didn't have to attend a function or some sort of get-together, I wouldn't. If it was something Channel 9 said was compulsory, or a thing with the family where Jamie-Lee was picking up an award at high school for example, I felt I had to go or I'd be shot. But there was some safety in that; I wasn't the one up on stage. The situations that made me feel a little wobbly were when I was talking to a group of people; if I had a seizure then and couldn't finish a sentence, or started speaking gibberish — that was the experience I feared. I can still remember being in conversation a couple of times when I was 99.99 per cent sure I didn't have one, but I used to think to myself after I delivered a sentence, 'That was the most stupid thing I've ever said; that didn't work properly.' I'd second guess myself and wonder, 'Did I get one and drop off the radar just briefly then?'

So I came close to being a social leper; didn't mix a lot with the neighbours and certainly not with friends as frequently as I used to. When it came to immediate family I had no real concerns because they knew about my epilepsy. It was things like attending parties or dinners that worried me more, as there was always the thought lingering in the back of my mind: 'I hope I don't have one here.'

I'm sure people thought I was either the quietest bloke in the world, or the most ignorant, when I'd stand in a group of people and not say a lot. I was always listening instead; it was easy to get through that with one or two-word answers. I'd always laugh with them; that was how I coped.

There was an episode just weeks before my on-air seizures in November 2006 that also acted as a strong indication that my life couldn't go on like it had been. We were at a café in Fortitude Valley in Brisbane having breakfast after having dropped Jamie-Lee off at the pool to prepare for a water polo match. After talking to the bloke who delivered the food to the table, I began to tuck into my bacon and eggs. All of a sudden I dropped my knife and fork and my head virtually dropped right into my breakfast plate. Another seizure had gripped me, and it was stronger than usual.

Jacqui grabbed my arm and walked me out of the café but I couldn't get my legs to work. When I reached the concrete strip in the car park (you know, the ones across the front of each car spot to stop you going any further forward), I tripped over it. My feet seemed to be dragging along the ground and Jacqui jumped under my arm to take the weight before loading me into the car. She took me home where I slept from about 10am to 3pm. Not long after that, when I had a minor seizure in the car when Jacqui was with me, it all came to a head.

Driving the car has become a challenge at times. On a few occasions, I felt a seizure coming on while in the car, but I'd be aware enough to pull over to the side of the road and wait until it had passed. Only once in my life behind the wheel — 32 years — did I get caught in a tense situation: it came only a few days before my on-screen meltdown.

Jacqui, Jamie-Lee and one of our nieces were in the car when I started to have a seizure behind the wheel. Jacqui could see it and screamed at me, 'Pull over! Pull over, Wally ... now!' She looked at me with that determined 'Now listen to me' look and said, 'That's it — you are not doing this any more. If it were just you or you and me in the car, that's fine; but not with the kids. You have to do something.'

She was right.

FIVE

TOUGH TIMES

THE period when my concern about my epilepsy and frequency of seizures grew just happened to coincide with an uneasy last few years of my football career. During that time, I was sacked from the Broncos captaincy, then dumped by the club altogether; had three seasons at the Gold Coast which ended in a fair bit of conflict between me and the club; and we discovered that Jamie-Lee was profoundly deaf. I can't say that period from late 1989 to 1993 was the most enjoyable of my life but it was certainly character building, although it was also a time when some friendships, or relationships, were stretched.

One of the things that troubled me most was Wayne Bennett's claim that I was not the right sort of person to be his captain any longer; I was unapproachable, according to other players, and didn't handle the media right. To be honest, that astounded me. Almost every day I spoke to at least one of the radio, newspaper or television outlets. It was normally a group interview after training where I was asked the usual questions: mostly my thoughts on the game just completed, my views on the game ahead and selections. Bennett suggested that it was just part of the captain's job, and while I concede dealing with the media is generally accepted as being one of a skipper's duties, I felt a certain touch of irony in his suggestions I didn't handle it well enough, considering that an interview with the coach was as rare as hen's teeth. I couldn't see why it was okay for him to distance himself from the media, and only talk to them after the Saturday morning training session, whilst being critical of my input.

He also declared he wanted a captain who wouldn't be away in the representative teams. His insistence that a player must be with his team every week was understandable, even if I didn't agree with it, but at that stage the Broncos had 10 players playing State of Origin and two more, Dale Shearer and Kevin Walters, joining us in 1990. That left Greg Dowling (who'd retired from rep football at the end of 1988), Brett Le Man and James Donnelly as regular first graders who weren't in the rep teams. Bennett asked Dowling to take over but 'GD' declined. I can recall talking to Gene Miles during a physiotherapy session we both attended prior to Dowling knocking the job back. Geno said, 'Gee, I'd hate to be in GD's shoes.' A couple of days later, it appeared those boots mightn't have been so uncomfortable after all.

Bennett had approached Gene and offered him the captaincy if he retired from representative football. Geno consulted me during another physio session and told me he'd been offered the position, but had been hesitant to accept and he just wanted to run it by me.

I told Gene I was confused: 'Why would he offer it to you when he's already declared it can't go to a representative player?' Geno's reply stunned me; he claimed that he was thinking about retiring from representative football immediately. This came just a day after we'd been talking about maybe making 1990 our last year at representative level, and a successful one at that, ending with the Kangaroo tour. Gene replied that he'd been thinking about calling it quits for a while. It seemed his plans had suddenly been altered following that meeting with Bennett.

I asked him if he agreed with Wayne's decision to drop me as captain and he said, 'No, not at all.' For me, that was enough. If you don't agree with something, it's pretty well impossible to pretend you do. Perhaps it was occurring in reverse (he did agree but was pretending not to), although Gene assured me that wasn't the case. To me, it was simple: if he did agree with the coach, then admit it and take the job; if he didn't, then knock it back. In the end, I said something like, 'Mate, if that's what you want, if you agree with what's been said, then you take it on.' I heard him announce at a press conference the following day that he had considered the role and then got back to me that morning to inform me he was accepting the position. I was filthy; let's just say we had a different interpretation about what transpired.

Geno and I didn't talk too much after that unless it was in the context of a team talk or during the game. I was pretty hurt by what had happened. If my best mate from football didn't agree with the change in captaincy, why did he crack? And if he had, why not tell me up front? It was hard enough to accept that I had lost the Brisbane captaincy when I was the Queensland and Australian captain, but Gene hopping in my grave made it more difficult to digest.

After one more season with the Broncos, I was dumped by Brisbane and went to the Gold Coast, and a year later, Gene went to play with Wigan in England, so we didn't see much of each other. In May 1992, his team was playing in the Challenge Cup final, the biggest game in England, and although it had been a while since we'd spoken, I thought I'd ring him and wish him the best. I called the Wigan football club on the morning of the game, and asked how I could get in contact with him. They gave me a hotel number in London, and after the receptionist transferred me to the room, I was expecting to leave a message. Gene answered and was obviously surprised I'd called. After the usual 'What's doing?' I said something like, 'I just wanted to wish you all the best; it's one match I never got to experience as I only had a brief time with Wakefield. I hope it goes well for you. Anyway, I know it's match day and you must have a heap of things to do, so I'll let you go. Good luck for the day, have a good one — enjoy it.'

Gene said he was in no rush, there wasn't a lot to do and we may as well keep talking. It was good to break the ice and we spoke for probably 45 minutes. During the conversation, Brisbane and Wayne Bennett came up, and how he had a habit of getting rid of older players a season early rather than a season too late. Gene laughed and said something about how he and Greg Dowling weren't retained by the club after completing contracts, and I'd know the difference when it came to the Broncos' official retirement announcements and the real story; that their parting wasn't quite as mutual as had been made out.

Bit by bit our friendship was restored, initially through the 'Godfather of Queensland State of Origin', Dick 'Tosser' Turner, because Maroons old boys organisation called FOGS (Former Origin Greats) was being set up; Gene is the executive director of the body now. But it took a while and neither of us would deny that it never got back to how it was previously — we were nearly inseparable for a long while.

The 1992 and 1993 seasons were fairly stressful and that was the period I was most troubled by seizures while involved in footy. I signed for the Gold Coast for the 1991 season amid a fair bit of fanfare, but we came last in the three seasons I was there, the last two when I was coach. All through my career I've been a pretty ordinary loser, but the Gold Coast record was particularly hard to swallow. All of the players gave their best on the field, and while I was determined to make them better footballers, there were several things that made that more difficult.

I'm not trying to dismiss any criticism of my coaching. I was very inexperienced, but I felt the difficulties the players and I were forced to deal with were ridiculous at times. For example, in 1993 we travelled to Wollongong to play the Illawarra Steelers, and I believed the boys were quite capable of chalking up a win. After arriving in Sydney around mid-afternoon, we boarded a bus to travel down the Princes Highway to Wollongong. The players appeared to be in a very confident state, but their mood was severely jolted upon our arrival in the 'Gong. The bus stopped at a caravan park, and at first the players laughed as they thought we'd been delivered to the wrong address. I joined the other officials and quizzed the driver, but we soon found that he'd brought us to the address given by the Seagulls club. Yep, we were to stay in a caravan park, most of us in some relocatable cabins. It caused instant fury amongst the players and severely affected any chance we had of winning the football match the next day. The players needed to be addressed as soon as possible, so a meeting was called and I centred on getting them to produce their best on the field as a perfect way to prove to the Seagulls' bosses that they should have been treated a little better.

At the close of the meeting, the coaching staff felt quite comfortable with the players' level of determination, and we decided to go to a hall where our dinners were to be served. Before we adjourned, the coaches and team managers had a quick meeting to discuss plans for the next day, but those plans were quickly thrown into disarray when we arrived at the hall to find that some of the players had been offered frozen meals that were to be heated in microwave ovens! If that wasn't enough to raise the players' fury, they soon discovered that the club officials were staying at the best hotel in town opposite the beach! All the players headed out to get their own dinners, with McDonald's or the local pizza place getting a workout.

It made the next day tough. We were determined to prove to the committee that a more professional approach was required, but the full-time scoreline failed to support our argument — we lost 26–0. If that terrible experience wasn't bad enough, the bus broke down on the way back to Sydney and we were forced to stay in Wollongong for an extra night.

When we returned to the Gold Coast, the players' — and the coaches' — dissatisfaction was made very clear. I met with Seagulls Leagues Club general manager Vic Folitarik, who hadn't been at the club long but seemed to be gunning for me from the start. However, he declared to me that I, and the players, had his full support. He suggested they be reminded that, as owners, the Tweed Heads Seagulls club fully backed the Gold Coast Seagulls team in the ARL premiership. I returned to the training session, which had just begun on the adjoining field, with a little extra spring in my step.

That soon disappeared. Just after the players took to the field to begin training, a group of journalists asked to speak to me briefly. One asked me what I thought about Folitarik's comments. I replied that they sounded great and he had our full support. That stunned the journalists, and they soon advised me that Folitarik had just delivered heavy criticism of me. Their claims left me a little confused, but all the media agreed that was definitely the case.

I headed back over to see Folitarik, and after I explained what I'd just been told, he began giggling before adding that the journalists must have misunderstood him. He assured me he'd said, 'There will be plenty of people suggesting that Wally has no idea about coaching, but it was important to prove to those people that he could, and the only way to do that was on the field.' I left feeling a little more comfortable.

Upon returning to the training paddock the journalists asked me if I'd fronted Folitarik. I replied that I had and, in fact, he'd guaranteed me his full support and claimed that the journos must have misunderstood him.

What happened next was startling. Almost as a team, the journos said, 'Well, you have a listen to what he said,' and they were all holding up their tape recorders, offering to provide the evidence. One pushed the 'play' button and I was left in no doubt that Folitarik had just lied to me. He virtually said that I had no idea about what I was doing and that the club had no faith in me.

I wheeled around and headed straight back to Folitarik's office, but he'd shut his door and refused to let me in. His secretary covered for him by saying he was on the phone, but from a side window it was obvious he wasn't — he was hiding from having to confront me as I yelled from his secretary's desk outside to open up and speak with me.

Days later, I had to front a board meeting where the events of the previous few days were discussed. There had been headlines about my poor relationship with Folitarik that only added further stress to the club, which had been suffering some financial instability. After entering the meeting it was obvious that the board fully supported the general manager; they claimed that while the event had been an unfortunate incident, there were still bright times ahead for the club. But after listening to the club's version of their plan for the future, I knew I had next to no support whatsoever, and the best thing to do for the players' sake was to call it quits.

Following my resignation, Folitarik was leaving the building when a good mate of mine, television journalist Glenn Palmer, approached him, but was ignored when he asked for a comment on my departure. Glenn then said, 'Why not give your side of the story — everyone has to listen to Lewis' side of the argument.' Folitarik wheeled around and said, 'Yes, yes, why not?'

Palmer asked one or two basic questions to which Folitarik gave his version of events, before Glenn — who had been researching Folitarik — raised some questions about his sudden departures from a couple of licensed clubs in Newcastle. Folitarik looked stunned and refused to answer any of the questions, which kept coming at him until he walked into his office and slammed the door in Glenn's face. The story ran on Channel 7 with comments from officials at the relevant clubs casting some aspersions on Folitarik's reign at their clubs.

While I was very sad to leave the Seagulls, a smile was brought to my face some weeks later with one of the players ringing to tell me that Folitarik was no longer with the club. I hoped the board members were having a little trouble swallowing that night.

In the middle of all the turmoil with the Gold Coast club, I also coached the Queensland State of Origin team in 1993, which was a great honour, and continued into 1994 before handing over the reins to Paul Vautin. That ended my association with rugby league in an 'official' capacity.

While I'll forever feel blessed for the experiences and achievements I was able to have in rugby league, I learned fairly dramatically in 1991 that nothing is more important than family — when we discovered, just before her first birthday, that Jamie-Lee was deaf. There had been one or two suspicions, but whenever we'd call her she seemed to respond immediately. There were times when she didn't, but neither did her two brothers sitting alongside her, so it became something we thought we'd imagined. We took her to the local doctor only to be informed that there didn't appear to be a problem; just a build-up of the flu. Of course, it was something I'd heard before in regard to my epilepsy, but I didn't become too worried.

However, when I dropped a dinner plate from the kitchen table one day, shattering it on the tiles, she was standing right alongside it but didn't react at all. The boys did, and they were about 8 to 10 metres away sitting on the balcony with the sound of breaking surf in the background.

We arranged a further hearing test and travelled to Brisbane, where the results revealed she had a massive build-up of fluid in her ears, so she underwent an operation to insert 'grommets', which are miniature tubes used to drain excess fluid from the ears. We were told that it would take around a week or so for the ears to clear. Then she'd come back to have them removed and be retested. Upon our return we had plenty of company; there were several other parents waiting for their children, who were undergoing the same 30-minute procedure.

After about 45 minutes, we made some comment about the operation seemingly taking a little longer than the others. There had been plenty of banter and exchanging of conversation in the waiting room, but when our wait stretched to 60 minutes, then 90, I started to fear the worst. I just knew something was wrong. But I didn't want to create panic for Jacqueline or her mother, who had come along hoping to be present for the good news. Just before the two-hour mark, a nurse approached and asked us to follow her down a long corridor. She asked us to sit down and wait for the doctor, and the look on her face told the story. It was gut wrenching. The doctor came out to explain how the procedure had gone and Jacqueline jumped in anxiously with, 'How's Jamie-Lee?' He declared, 'Yes, she's fine … but, well … there is …'

It seemed he couldn't finish the sentence. As Jacqueline went to inquire again, he took a deep breath and said, 'I'm sorry but your daughter is profoundly deaf.' I'd never heard the term 'profoundly' used before, but before I got a chance to ask for the medical definition Jacqueline jumped in with, 'Will she be able to hear anything?' The reply cut right through us: 'I'm sorry, no.'

Jacqueline collapsed on the ground and I wasn't much better, but felt I had to listen to the doctor's description of the testing that Jamie-Lee had gone through. He couldn't look me in the eye. It must be one of the hardest things for our wonderful doctors to do — to inform the family of sad news or tragedy. I don't remember a single word he said — I was in shock.

It was a moment of trauma we'll never ever forget; but, as we have come to understand, Jamie-Lee has gone on with her life in an admirable way and never sought sympathy. She regards herself as just like anybody else in the street, and while she has been robbed of one of the necessities of life others take for granted, there are plenty of times she has considered herself lucky that she doesn't have to listen to her mother's and father's continual requests.

The news arrived at a very difficult time. It was the day before the deciding game of the 1991 State of Origin series at Lang Park, and I was captaining Queensland. After being delivered the bad news, I headed to Lang Park. I'd asked coach Graham Lowe if I could get there a little late for the final training session, but because we'd been so long at the hospital, I arrived just as the session was finishing. Our manager 'Tosser' Turner, who was aware of the reason for my absence, took one look at me and knew what must have happened. He walked over to Lowe, spoke to him, and all of a sudden the training session restarted. But it was a waste of time; my mind was somewhere else and I couldn't concentrate on the ball or the upcoming game. Rugby league had always been such a big part of my life; in fact, Jacqueline would probably argue that on some occasions it meant more to me than anything else. That changed that day.

Prior to kickoff the next evening, I called Tosser aside to tell him, 'This is it.' I'd decided there were much more important things in life than footy. Later, Tosser told me that if I hadn't made that decision he would have suggested it, albeit leaving it until after full-time. Thankfully, Queensland won the match 14–12, Mal Meninga kicking the only goal of the game from wide-out to convert a try by Dale Shearer, ensuring all three matches of that series were won by two points. My retirement from Origin was announced before full-time and I took Mitchell and Lincoln around that great stadium for a farewell lap after the game. It was another experience from a couple of days I won't forget.

SIX

JACQUELINE

YOU'VE probably gathered by now that Jacqueline has been a shining light in my life; she is the bubbly, talkative one who is quick to throw her emotions out there for everyone to see but who, I'd imagine, wouldn't have an enemy in the world.

I'm sure I see more humour in it than Jacqueline does, but there is a funny story around how we came into each other's lives. It was Nobbys Beach on the Gold Coast in 1983, and it happened thanks to a mate of mine from the surf club, Mark Wilson.

'Willo' played football with my younger brothers Edwin and Scott and I'd known him just about all my life. Anyway, Mark started going out with this girl Kayleen (they're now married) and I thought it must have been getting a little serious, because Willo didn't normally stick with one girl longer than a couple of dates. Now all the boys, as boys do, were glowing in their praise of Kayleen's well-rounded figure … and her personality.

When I was introduced to Kayleen, she was with her sister, Jacqueline Green. I must say, both were very attractive young ladies. Anyway, to cut a long story short I took a shine to Jacqui instantly and soon after asked her out. But she'd been going through a break-up with another bloke and wasn't interested. I kept running into her at the surf club, though, and did my best to win her over. Eventually, I convinced her to go out for dinner and, while it went well, it ended as quickly as it began — with not even a kiss! I did get her to come to lunch the odd time but she didn't want to 'go out' with me. Soon after, she said she was going to try to get back with her former boyfriend and see how it went.

But I was a persistent bastard. At the time, I owned a deli/lunch bar with my mother called the Rhine Barrel at the K-Mart shopping complex at Cannon Hill, often starting my day with an early-morning trip to the fish markets to join the auction for the best seafood available. I enjoyed working with the old lady, except for cutting the ham; I could never cut enough of it, it seemed. In the complex was a florist and, to win over Jacqui's heart, I'd send her flowers every few days, hoping she'd come around. I remember the florist saying to me one day, 'Mate, if this bird won't go out with you after all these flowers, at least you're keeping me in business!' I sent her five dozen carnations for her 21st birthday in September 1983 and gave her a diamond pendant, but she still wouldn't budge.

I went to see Jacqui at her house one evening and told her I had a couple of tickets to see David Bowie who was playing at Lang Park, but she said she had other plans for the night. I thought, 'Stuff it,' so I asked another girl out and when we arrived home from the concert there was Jacqui parked outside — and I had another woman in the car!

She said, 'Can I talk to you please … who's that?' I explained, 'It's the girl I just went out with; you said you wouldn't — remember? What are you here for?' She said she'd changed her mind. So I, quite rudely the other girl would have thought, ordered a taxi to take her home and Jacqui came inside and we had a good talk.

There were plenty of hurdles still to negotiate. I'd only been back a week or two from the Queensland team's tour of England and just the day before I'd agreed to return for a brief stint with the Wakefield Trinity club. I thought, 'Shit, I finally get a breakthrough with Jacqui and I'm taking off overseas.'

After touring with the 1982 Kangaroos and then going back for the Queensland tour straight after the Brisbane season had finished, to be honest, I really wanted a summer at home. But a guy called Barry Hough at Wakefield was more persistent in getting me to agree to play for the club than I was in trying to get Jacqui to go out with me. I was determined not to go — it didn't really interest me too much while I was trying to become 'an item' with Jacqui. But her decision to try again with the former boyfriend tempted me to go; and the club agreed for my brother Scott, who was also playing first grade for Valleys, to come with me. You couldn't believe the timing of it all.

Signing for Wakefield is another funny story that I should mention. During the Queensland tour, Leeds had approached me to come back to the UK for a short stint before the 1984 Australian season began, and were prepared to pay me £500 a match. But I wasn't particularly interested and told them to contact me after I got home, just to put them off until I left. Someone from Wakefield also rang me before I left England, but I also told them I wasn't interested.

Not long after I got back to Brisbane, Barry, a millionaire supporter of Wakefield Trinity, rang me and asked what I'd want to entice me to play for them until the start of the Aussie season. I told him I wasn't interested, but he rang back the next night and again the next night and said, 'We're prepared to offer you £300 a game.' Barry's original offer was £160, then £180, before he bumped it up to £250. In those days the English pound was only worth $1.27, and travelling to the other side of the world for $317 a week was hardly enticing.

Barry said, 'We're going to be having a board meeting early tomorrow morning and you can let us know then.' I said, 'Mate, I'm telling you I don't want to go.'

He called again the following night and told me he was in the boardroom with the club directors and said the board had agreed to pay his suggested match fee of £400. I replied that that wasn't a lot of money, especially with the exchange rate being so low; I still wasn't interested. He upped it to £500 a game, then after a few more refusals £650, and I could hear the committeemen in the background saying, 'Bloody 'ell, we won't be paying *thart* much *mooney*.'

I was unmoved and was about to hang up when Barry said, 'You give us your final figure, and if we can't meet it we can officially say no and that will be that.' I said, 'If you want me over there, you'll have to double that (the £650 match fee to £1300), plus I want two return airfares for my brother Scott and me. We want to stay at a good hotel — it doesn't have to be the Hilton or the Sheraton but a comfortable place to stay for such a long period. We also want a car to drive around.' Scott was paid the basic match payments of, I think, £115 a win and £15 a loss.

I could hear all the blokes screaming and carrying on in the background, and I said, 'There you go, that's the end of that.' You could have blown me over when Barry said, quick as a flash, 'Done. There's a plane leaving Thursday. Be on it; I'll be at the airport to pick you up!' I couldn't believe it. I didn't want to go and I told him, 'Mate, I want to stay here in the off-season,' but he claimed we'd agreed to terms and I was obligated. I thought this bloke might sue me now if I didn't go. Then I thought, well, Jacqui won't go out with me, there was nothing particularly keeping me at home, it will only be for a few weeks, so …

That was the night before Jacqui came around and said she'd changed her mind about going out with me. Geez, I was in a real pickle now. I'd agreed to play 10 matches for Wakefield Trinity, I'd committed Scott — who was 19 — to go with me before I'd even asked him (as it turned out, he was happy to make the trip), and I hadn't mentioned anything to the Queensland Rugby League who wouldn't have been happy with me risking injury by playing in England. Surprisingly, Ron McAuliffe, the QRL Chairman and most powerful figure in Queensland rugby league, ended up giving me his blessing, provided that an injury insurance policy was in place.

After I signed the deal with Wakefield, I demanded that under no circumstance were they to mention how much money I was being paid, as it would cause dissension in the playing ranks. They agreed but needn't have bothered … the day I flew into Leeds Bradford airport, on the back page of the *Yorkshire Post* was a story saying 'Aussie gets £1000 per game'. Luckily they didn't know I was actually getting £1300! Barry had decided to pay the extra £300 out of his own pocket without the board knowing; they did think I was getting £1000. He was a wonderful bloke who I spent plenty of time with, and, as is so often the case in the UK, his whole life revolved around his favourite sports club.

When I got to training the only players who'd shake my hand were Australians — Brad Waugh from Penrith and Allan Burns from North Sydney. The irony was that in my first match for Wakefield, I came up against Peter Sterling, who was the big signing for Hull. After the scores were 16-all at half-time, we ran out of steam and lost 32–16. But after that the players finally came around as they could see Scott and I were having a real dig and, other than their cold welcome for the first few weeks, I thoroughly enjoyed my time at Wakefield and I'm glad I had the opportunity to play in the English league for the only time in my career.

I'd left for the UK a few days after Jacqui finally decided I was worthy of going out with her, and I was keen for her to come over for a few weeks to join me. One problem was that she'd had holiday leave from her work not long before; but the bigger trouble was getting her old man to agree to it.

Her father Bruce, who I get on with famously well, was a tough old wharfie. I'll never forget the first time I went to Jacqui's place at Hawthorne in Brisbane and we were introduced. He was lying on the lounge watching television and I said, 'G'day, Bruce, how you going?' and went to shake hands. He had his hands behind his head, with a toothpick in his mouth, stretched back on the couch and just nodded without saying a word. Jacqui's mother Kathy said, 'Bruce, don't be so rude; you were just introduced,' and he replied, 'I said g'day,' and just kept watching TV.

Jacqui then intervened and said, 'Dad, I've just introduced you,' and he said, looking towards me, 'I'll be honest; I don't like you.' Great start! The bloke was dirty on me before we'd even met; an event I was looking forward to ended up an uncomfortable nightmare.

The first thing I did to get Jacqui to come over to England was call her boss in the smallgoods factory where she worked in a secretarial role and ask if he'd allow her to go on holidays for a couple of weeks. He was hesitant, so I told him I owned a delicatessen and if he let her come over, we'd buy all our hams off his company, KR Dowling Downs. He agreed.

With the first hurdle navigated I called Jacqui, who was still reluctant to make the trip, and told her it was all clear with her boss. She said her father was still the biggest barrier, but she'd talk to him, and he ended up saying she could go. By this time I was in England and then she told me that when she thought more about it, she couldn't afford it anyway. I said, 'Go and see my mother at lunchtime.' So she went to our lunch bar and told my mum that I'd asked her over to England. Mum said, 'Yeah, I know … Wally asked me to give you this.' She opened up an envelope and inside was a plane ticket. I called the deli number while Jacqui was there and explained that she had no excuse to say no now. She came over with Scott's girlfriend Terri just after Christmas.

I guess you could say it was love at first sight, for one of us at least, and I didn't muck around much when I realised Jacqui was the woman for me. While she was in England, in early January, I bought an engagement ring and proposed, and luckily she said 'yes'. We'd known each other for probably four months and been going out for just 16 days — and for 12 of those, I'd been in England.

I thought I'd call Bruce myself to make sure he was comfortable with our big decision. I was nervous and said,

'G'day, Bruce, you know how Jacqui and I have been going out for a while and …' He jumped in with, 'I wouldn't call 16 days a long time.' That only increased the heart rate further and I meekly replied with, 'No, no … I don't suppose it is.' I kept up some nervous small-talk and was stalling when he said, 'Well, what can I do for you?'

I thought, Stuff it, here goes. 'Anyway, Bruce, I wanted to do the right thing, as old fashioned as it might be these days, and ask the father for his daughter's hand in marriage. I've already asked Jacqui and she said yes.' He said, 'Oh well, if she said yes, there's not much I can do; it's up to her.' I thought, How good's this! I'd thought I was 1000 to 1 of getting his blessing; well, kind of a blessing.

We were married on 10 November 1984, having just bought our first home together (I'd owned one previously at Holland Park) in a suburb called Norman Park, a renovated Queenslander and the type of house I always wanted, with 270 degree views. One of the things I ensured we discussed before we got married was what Jacqui was taking on in the role of being the partner of a high-profile footballer. I told her the phone would run off the hook, our lives would be played out in the media, people would interrupt us when we were in public wanting an autograph or a chat and she'd have to be a wife, secretary, spokesperson and representative to the media; but she said she was fine with that. After about 18 months of married life, by which time she was well pregnant with Mitchell, she must have been wondering what she'd got herself into.

Despite the drastic changes that soon became part of her life, Jacqui remained very much the same person. She's always been very patient; she definitely has her views on issues and doesn't mind voicing them. But there was one thing that was going to have to change, as marrying a bloke from Valleys, the team her family — Easts supporters — despised, meant she might have to support a team she never had before. But the changes never seemed to cause any dramas and she was quite comfortable with our lifestyle. She's been a wonderful partner to have — through good times and in bad, through sickness and in health. She's had plenty of all that.

SEVEN

THE KIDS

Jacqui and I could not have wished to have been blessed with three more wonderful children. It's not always easy having a parent who is well known publicly (well, Lincoln is quite recognisable too now in his own right through his role on the television serial *Home and Away*), but they've handled that well and each forged their own goals in life and shown a great work ethic and determination in everything they've pursued.

Mitchell was born on 30 April 1986, Lincoln on 24 October 1987 and Jamie-Lee on 7 June 1990. As a family, I'd like to think we're very close and the boys have been wonderful to their little sister; Mitch particularly when she was younger, and naturally felt a bit lonely, with few kids wanting to play with a girl who was deaf. Mitchell used to take her to the movies on the days they had subtitles on the screen even if he'd seen it two or three times before. They used to have fun; he'd tell us how she reacted to the show and if she didn't pick up something, he'd explain it to her along the way, although every now and then she'd tell him to shut up.

For years Mitch has worked at a cinema in Hawthorne, now as a manager, and he loves the production side of movies and the media. He's always wanted to be behind the camera, while from a young age Lincoln wanted to be in front of it as an actor. Mitch, who has a wonderful easy-going chatty temperament like his mother, began working at the cinema part-time at night for extra money while he was still at school. He still works there part-time but also has a job as assistant producer for the breakfast program at Nova FM in Brisbane, which he reckons is the flashest name ever for 'coffee go-getter'; but he loves it.

So these days he works early in the morning at Nova, starting at 5.30am and finishing at about noon, for not much money (which is standard in radio for those type of positions); gets a bit of a snooze during the day, then is off to the cinema to work at night. I've inquired at Channel 9 about a job as a cameraman in television, but he honestly enjoys the radio work at Nova so much that at this stage I think he's in no hurry to change. He has his own gig on the show doing his weekly movie review which he loves; they call it 'The Right Royal Movie Review'. He's keen on his snow skiing too and other than his regular trips to Thredbo, he travelled to Japan for the first time in 2008 on a skiing trip.

What I would never do is push the kids into any sport; being the offspring of a well-known sportsperson brings its own problems, without them being reluctant in the first place. Mitch loved his footy from the days when he first turned out for the Burleigh Bears.

Generally he was pretty tough and had a lot of passion for his footy. He did come up against the odd abuse because he was my son; one day the father of an opposing player was into him savagely, yelling continual abuse — this was under-7s! He later played hooker and kept playing until he was 15. He was much more like his mother — if he lost, it was a case of, 'Oh well, I wish we'd won today but so and so did this right; these blokes did that well; the kid on the other team was very good at doing this.' He'd assess the game for what it was and accepted they weren't good enough this time.

Lincoln was more like me if his team was beaten: absolutely filthy. Linc had quite a bit of talent as a footballer and while he enjoyed the hard side of it, that's not the way he began. We travelled from the Gold Coast to Ipswich — a distance of about 110 kilometres — to watch him play his first match for the Burleigh Bears at six years of age.

He had quite a cheer squad that day, with his grandparents joining Jacqueline and me on the sidelines to cheer him on. But after running onto the field, Lincoln had to be carried off before kick-off; he'd gone down with 'bindies' or prickles in his foot. Despite this setback, he always had this real determined look on his face when he ran the ball or went in for a tackle.

When he went into full-field footy he played centre and was a little like me; his comfort always seemed to be controlled by the match result. For a couple of years I believed Lincoln probably felt compelled to reach greater heights, but I made sure he understood that he was under no pressure at all, and that he should continue to play only if he wanted to. Jacqueline and I had always stressed that if they wanted to try something else, go with the flow. And of course, growing up can be difficult; there are lots of other things that teenage boys become interested in!

Eventually, when he got to under-18 level, a lot of his mates had changed to rugby union. He followed them and played centre and wing. Unfortunately, he fell into some of the rah-rah traits — like diving like an Olympic gymnast for a try. One day we went to see him play for his new club Easts, and with his grandparents, Jacqueline and I sitting behind the goalposts at the city end of the field, he scored a 60-metre runaway try and he almost dived over the cross bar putting the ball down — it was almost like it was a competition between him and his mates. Didn't I give it to him!

Linc was probably five or six when he said he wanted to be an actor; it was a 'garbo' before that. We thought wanting to be on TV was natural at that age, and he'd grow out of it; but he never changed his mind. And it's a great reward for his determination and resilience that he now has his part as Geoff Campbell on *Home and Away*.

He won a few TV commercial roles when he was in his teens, including ones for Dreamworld, Australia Post, Kingston Park Raceway and Nutri-Grain. I'll never forget the time I had to take him down to the Gold Coast for an audition for a Nutri-Grain commercial and he had to take his push bike to do some tricks on. It didn't fit into the boot, so I had to loosen the handle bars and twist it at all angles to get the damn thing in the car. We ended up tearing the upholstery and scratching paint off the door as it went in. Anyway, we got down there and he had to ride down a big hill straight at the cameras. The directors said they were looking for kids who could ride bikes well and do some stunts and asked Lincoln if he could do that. 'Sure,' he said, although he wasn't particularly confident or comfortable on a bike, let alone flying down a steep hill and doing tricks. I said, 'Are you sure about that?' and he replied, 'Well, I couldn't tell them I wasn't great at riding a bike.'

The first kid flew down the hill from about 30 metres, lifted high in the air and came down and did a big wheel stand. Then he went down a further 70 or 80 metres, before applying the front brakes so he was on the front wheel only. He raced down, stood up on his bike while it was in the air, and everyone was clapping, saying what a genius he was; he added a few tricks as well. The next boy went arse over head, as did the third, fourth, fifth and sixth.

Lincoln had his first turn and crashed down the bottom of the hill and flew over the handle bars. He explained that, seeing as we had to adjust the brakes so much to get the bike into the car, they were a bit touchy, and asked for another go. He came down the second time, went into the air and landed safely, went again and hit the brake and flew down probably 10 metres just on the front wheel. The director said, 'Good — that was terrific.' I said to Lincoln, 'How the hell did you do that?' and he honestly had no idea. I could say that the old Lewis determination just came out of him somehow, but we'd both admit it was a fluke at best. Anyway, he got the part. It was the first of a few commercials he ended up doing; it was his big start.

Lincoln was fortunate to land roles in two movies too — *Aquamarine* and *Voodoo Lagoon* (as one of the lead characters) — and was a presenter on the TV show *Kids Biz*, but *Home and Away* has certainly been his big break. In *Voodoo Lagoon* he performed with ex-*Home and Away* star Beau Brady, *Neighbours* star Natalie Blair and the girl who won the first series of *It Takes Two*, Erica Heynatz, who he had to do a love scene with.

Unfortunately, he'd just missed out on two previous roles on *Home and Away* — once for the role of Ric and the other time for Drew. When he didn't get the second role, he was shattered and when he auditioned for Geoff Campbell he was pretty nervous, thinking it might be his last shot. His mother was always egging him on, saying, 'Keep going, that's okay, they must think you're good to keep calling you back.' He was shopping with his mother one day when his phone rang. The next thing, he screamed out and everyone around them jumped, then stared. He'd just been advised he'd got the part.

Before joining *Home and Away*, he'd worked as a fitness instructor at first, working in gymnasiums and as a personal trainer; he really enjoyed it and became very interested in it. But his greatest passion has always been acting.

The irony was that the biggest moment in his acting career coincided with the biggest moment in regard to my health; he auditioned for the part on *Home and Away* in Melbourne just a few kilometres away from where I sat in hospital undergoing tests to decide my suitability for brain surgery. Fortunately, we both had a positive outcome.

Lincoln has worked hard to get a television role and continues to work hard; hearing his stories when he comes home some weekends has given me an appreciation of what actors go through at times on those serials. He can have some light days where he might only be on the set for an hour and has to sit around for a few hours before he's required again for another hour or so then not have any filming for a couple of days; other times he can be on the set most of the day and into the night. And there are the rehearsals and memorising the scripts, so there is a lot of work off screen. But the point that amazed me throughout was his ability to memorise the scripts; something that had become absolutely impossible for his old man during the past few years.

I don't think a lot of people understand the hours that actors put into it so that they can recall a scene and be able to speak without any interruptions and portray it with the right body movement, face, and to have genuine character about it. It's been a real eye opener to me talking to Lincoln about what is involved and I have a great respect for the profession.

Probably the most difficult part is when they film in winter but it's made out to be a nice, warm summer day.

In fact it's made out to be beautiful comfortable surroundings 12 months of the year; they hardly seem to have a rainy or overcast day in Summer Bay! One time he had to do a couple of the bush scenes, being a boy from the country, where he had to sprint down a hill towards his pop who didn't know who he was and fired a gun, which caused Lincoln to fall and slide in the wet grass. Lincoln said it was bloody freezing and they were still filming at 10.30 at night and it got to the stage where he thought, 'Surely they're happy with that take,' only for him to be asked to do it again. He ended up getting a bit of the flu but you don't get sick days off with tight television schedules; they just say they'll shoot that scene later in the week.

I must admit, originally I had little interest in *Home and Away*. If I was reading the news that night, it was quite usual for me to arrive home at about 7.25pm, or at about 7pm if I was just reporting for the day, and everybody in the household would be glued to the television watching *H & A*. I'd collect my dinner from the kitchen bench and shuffle off into another room with barely a 'hello'. But during my lengthy post-operation recovery period, I have to confess I watched the show every night. Some of my mates got a dig in and said that I fitted in quite well … that only people with half a brain watch the show!

And Linc has also had to learn to be a public figure, something I had to go through at a similar age — and that's not always easy. But it has its funny side, though. Lincoln moved into a unit at Dee Why when he first got the part in 2007, in a block that had about 30 units in it. There were a heap of big Pacific Islanders living there, most looking like bulky rugby league or rugby union props who probably worked part-time as bouncers in the local nightclubs or as labourers on building sites. On one of the first days there Lincoln was walking back to his unit and there was this group of blokes hanging around; one said to him, 'What you looking at, bro?' He shit himself, felt real intimidated and said something like, 'Nothing, mate; it's cool.'

Anyway, wherever he walked he felt these piercing eyes following him and was wondering what the hell he had done to get offside with them and whether they were going to give him a flogging. A few weeks later this one bloke said to him, 'Hey, come here, bro … you on *Home and Away*?' Lincoln was a bit guarded but said, 'Yeah I'm one of the actors on the show.' The big bloke called over some of his mates and smiled, 'Oh yeah, Jeff Campbell, right? Yeah, you're good, man, I like your part.' He found out they all were religious watchers of *Home and Away*; they thought the sun shone out of his arse after that and he'd get greeted with high fives and they'd always be asking him what happened next on the show. Ironically they were also keen to 'look after' Lincoln if any unwelcome faces were to appear, and they told him, 'Eh, bro, we're here to watch your back, anytime.' Linc got a good laugh out of it and enjoyed their friendship. He was there for nearly two years and loved it but moved a bit further up the coast into a rented house with a nice look over the ocean.

Mitch and Linc have always been real close as brothers, similar in some ways but very different in others. Linc is a bloke who ensures everyone is well aware of what his thoughts and feelings are. He gets out of bed with a smiling face every day and, if he comes downstairs and sees me sitting grumpily on a kitchen chair, he'll kiss me on the top of my thin-haired skull and say, 'What's happening, King?' He's very much like his mother in that he doesn't mind a chat and has definite opinions on things. But when his brother opens his mouth, Lincoln remains quiet, almost as a mark of respect. They stick up for each other, and believe in each other, and as a father that's terrific to see.

So too is the respect they have for their sister. Mitch and Linc are both well aware that Jamie-Lee was the one in the family born with the sports genes, but it's the level of determination she possesses that attracts their greatest respect.

Finding that Jamie-Lee was profoundly deaf was a shock to us, naturally. But she has never offered it as an excuse for failure to achieve and regards herself as just like anybody else in the street. She gets great support from her brothers, as well as from all her family and friends.

It is just wonderful to see Jamie-Lee living such a full life despite her deafness and that is a tribute to her attitude and the support she gets around her. The best decision we made was to follow the path of a cochlear implant for her — even though it caused some controversy at the time and put us under pressure from the deaf community.

Choosing the correct path for our daughter was an interesting period in our lives. It took us quite some time to decide Jamie-Lee's future, because we were determined to assess *all* of the options available and receive advice from experts in the field. And the advice from one of them proved very beneficial. Dimity Dornan was a well-respected speech therapist who was assisting a couple of hearing impaired children. She was just getting underway and had to work from her husband Peter's physiotherapy centre, using his office or one of the unused booths for consultations. She told us she could only treat four children at a time, and with all four positions filled, it might be impossible to help Jamie-Lee. I promised Dimity that if she treated my daughter, I'd help her get into a much bigger building where she could treat as many children as she wanted. And after several fundraising events, including a charity football match I arranged, Dimity moved into a former church that now provides a beautiful background for the children attending from all around Queensland. Dimity has a group of wonderful staff who assist the kids, and more Hear and Say centres have opened across the state.

It wasn't always smooth sailing for us, however. For a couple of years Jacqueline and I discussed the best way forward for Jamie-Lee, but to be honest we were always going to be guided by the experts. After two-and-a-half years of deliberation, we decided to go ahead and give our daughter the best chance of being able to hear. We had been in constant communication with Dimity, our family doctor John Craven, and her specialist and surgeon Dr Bruce Black. A cochlear implant was inserted and two weeks later it was officially switched on. It left Jacqui and me in tears when she reacted to sound for the first time. It also brought the family even closer, with Mitchell and Lincoln talking to her and getting some reaction, although Lincoln's patience was nothing compared to his older brother's; Linc would walk off after a short while to entertain himself elsewhere.

While we were ecstatic over the progress she was making, we became targets of several people from the deaf community who believed we didn't have the right to 'make' her hear. We were heavily criticised and were forced to defend ourselves on a *60 Minutes* debate on the subject after being accused of being 'butchers'. The deaf community believed we had no right making the decision for our daughter, and claimed, in fact, that we (the hearing) were 'the unlucky people of the world'.

We ended the discussion on a pretty good note. After being asked, 'Well, what if your daughter doesn't want to hear? What will she do? As you two seem to have made the decision for her, she has no choice,' Jacqui ended the argument by saying, 'Yes she does … if she doesn't want to be bothered by sound, she can simply switch it off!' It was a knock-out punch that seemed to dumbfound our 'opposition'.

Jamie-Lee had her first cochlear implant in January 1995 when she was four and a half, and she, and we, have had no regrets. She had a much more efficient and smaller implant 'update' in April 2006, about a centimetre by half a centimetre in size, placed into the skull just behind the ear. It was much less invasive and obvious than her first one, which required a cut from the side of her temple all the way around to about 5 centimetres behind her ear, in a semi-circle around the base of her hairline. By the way, when she first saw the cut required for my surgery, she declared to her mother, 'Mine is worse than his!'

Jamie-Lee attended St Anthony's Catholic school in Alexandra Hills and adapted quite well, although she was obviously behind her peers initially. She always loved sport, even if it meant she had to wear head gear at netball to prevent the implants being bumped. Jacqui says Jamie-Lee is a carbon copy of me in that she's so determined: 'She's just like you used to be, driving away from a football game; you refused to talk about the game if you lost, didn't want to know about it, didn't want to talk to anyone, just filthy on the world.' Jamie-Lee's competitive instincts just switch on when it comes to sport, but beyond that she's fairly placid and very kind-hearted.

She speaks her mind, though; calls a spade a spade — she'll let people know her opinion and it doesn't matter who they are; grandparents, brothers, friends or family friends, she puts her cards on the table. Being deaf, it can be a little difficult for her to comprehend things at times and communicating took a lot longer for her as she was growing up. Other times, it can be quite an advantage, like when she turns her hearing aid off when she's exhausted and in need of rest.

She's 19 now and is doing a TAFE course in Brisbane, studying fitness and coaching. She wants to be involved in sport but I don't know which way it will go, although I certainly encourage that, because she loves it. She currently coaches a water polo team at her former school, All Hallows, and has secured a premiership for them in the girls' first year. I'd love to see her work with deaf kids too, helping them adjust to having the cochlear implant.

Until my on-screen meltdown and decision to have the surgery, I never spoke about my epilepsy with the kids, as I didn't want to burden them with any of my concerns or insecurities. I'm fortunate that I never had a seizure in front of any of them. If I was at home and had some warning, I'd go into another room and tell them I was going for a lie-down or just not say anything, because I was determined they wouldn't witness what I might go through. My attitude was that 90 per cent of the general population didn't know what epilepsy was all about, so two young fellows going to high school were going to struggle to understand it, let alone their little sister, so I didn't want to push it down their throats.

As I've already said, Jacqueline obviously told them enough for them not to panic and to be aware of what was happening if I did ever have a seizure in their presence. Jacqui obviously had to teach herself how to deal with those situations; although she used to fire questions at me with all good intentions of helping me, they used to drive me crazy. In later times she was far more calm and quiet, thank God.

That was one of the bonuses of my certain strand of epilepsy — usually I'd get a brief warning that a seizure was coming on. If I thought, 'Christ, I have to get out of here,' I'd go into one of the bathrooms or lie down on the bed. It's strange talking about it now; you try to come up with your own theories, and one of mine was that when I went and lay down and closed my eyes, it never came on as seriously as at other times because I wasn't seeing anything; the brain wasn't reacting to anything that was in front of me, vision-wise.

Sometimes the kids would come in after I'd had a seizure and I'd still be lying there, just looking tired as far as they could make out. I don't think they ever witnessed slurred speech or anything that would have alarmed them.

That's why it was such a shock for them when I broke down on television, as well as when they found out all the details afterwards of how badly the epilepsy had affected me. Lincoln certainly didn't seem to handle it too well. Mitchell, as the eldest, was the one Jacqui had called on a fair bit over the years, so it wasn't such a shock to him.

At the time, Lincoln was very determined to get his acting career off to a good start and was involved in arranging his audition for a role on *Home and Away* when my first embarrassing gaffe on TV happened, so he didn't see it. Mitchell wasn't home either and didn't witness it, but he would have been told by plenty of people around him. To be honest, I don't think Jamie-Lee would have recognised the problem; she was probably watching *The Simpsons*!

The second time, the worst time, they were all home and saw it live on television. That hit them all very hard. Lincoln must have asked me three times on the car trip home that night if everything was still alright, so you could tell he was churning inside pretty badly. I answered him with, 'Mate, I'm fine, I'm good now but I've just got to see a doctor about this.' We'd never ever discussed the fact I had epilepsy until then.

The fact is that my role as a father and a husband diminished a little bit, because I always felt I might have a turn at any minute and I'd lost a lot of confidence when we went out as a family in public. A few times, we'd have a family function on and I'd opt out of it; I just feared that, if I went, there was half a chance I'd have a spasmodic attack and I'd embarrass them. I know they would have been happy to come to my aid or take me out of sight of other people, or more appropriately out of the conversation with other people, and I didn't want them to have to do that. It got fairly difficult for a little while. Certainly, if I only went out because they'd pressured me, and something then happened, they'd believe they only had themselves to blame. That's a stupid way to think about it, but I just preferred that if I was going to have an episode, it wouldn't be in their company.

Jacqui sometimes used to have a go about me not going out; I think in the end she understood there was a fair reason behind it. Ultimately, she probably felt a little more comfortable to be able to go to those functions, particularly school ones with Jamie-Lee, and just be able to relax in the company, and not have to be concerned with my health if I was there.

I felt a lot safer in my own armchair at home in the lounge room watching a bit of TV, that's for sure. Most nights I was happy just putting my feet up; even if I didn't get to sleep, if I just sort of relaxed, and had the eyes closed for a while, I would feel a lot more comfortable. It was my way of ensuring my brain wasn't getting a bit stressed.

EIGHT

THIS IS YOUR LIFE

IT was Sunday morning, 21 April 2002, and I was told I had to go to Channel 9 in Brisbane to do a promotion for the station, my employer, with news anchors Bruce Paige and Heather Foord. The location was on top of Mount Coot-tha overlooking the city centre — a lovely setting.

We did a few shots and the producer seemed happy, when we got the familiar call, 'Just one more.' I said to the cameraman that the most amusing thing when you're doing TV is how many times you hear 'one more time', but it never is the last time. Anyway, we did another shoot and I heard a voice, which at first I thought was Pagey having a joke, say, 'You have to do it again,' and I reacted with 'Yeah, I know; one more time!' I quickly thought, 'That wasn't Pagey,' and turned around to see Mike Munro standing there. He smiled and said, 'One more time, Wally,' then walked towards me and delivered those familiar lines ... 'Wally Lewis, this is your life.'

I pleaded that I was due to cover a rugby league match that afternoon, but Mike assured me I'd been excused. I went back to the Channel 9 studios where I had to wait for a couple of hours before the show would begin. I had a late breakfast and some coffee, and rang Jacqui with the old, 'Good one, you — you got me. How long have you known?'

I was kept apart from the arriving guests until the show started and I remember walking out and seeing a heap of friends, family, former team-mates, and even mates I grew up with. It was great, I was really appreciative of them coming and I was excited about catching up with them later; if not about the shit some of them were obviously about to dump on me in front of the camera.

They began filming and after insights from my parents, other family and early mates, it got onto my football career. *Uh oh*, I could feel it build inside of me. I thought, 'Oh no, here it comes ... oh shit ... not here, not now.' I was trapped.

Mike mentioned an incident in 1980 when I was choking with a laryngeal spasm after copping an elbow to the throat from Mark Graham playing for Valleys. Vision of me choking on the ground went up on the screen. Mike asked me about it and I couldn't get a sentence out. I started to talk but knew I was gone. I had to say something, but the same old cloud came over my body and whatever came out was absolute gibberish.

Those confusing next few moments went like this:

'Oooh … err … I don't know … I can see the way they're trying to … I don't know …'

Mike Munro: 'I think you copped an elbow in the throat and your larynx was crushed …'

'Yeah.'

'Do you remember that?'

'Yeah, but I get by with the players that only play, who only play … on the inside … uumm … I'm trying to work a way that's going to be on the … err.'

It was incredibly embarrassing. Gene Miles, Mal Meninga and Trevor Gillmeister came on stage and Mike asked them about the old times when we were playing. Whatever the boys said attracted a laugh from the audience but I was still not completely with it. As they walked off stage, Mike signalled a commercial break and we had an interlude — of five minutes, I suppose. I sat there thinking, 'Well, the day you feared has just come. At least it wasn't live to air, but it was in front of family and your best friends.'

I remember a bloke saying to me before we went back into recording, 'You right? Everything okay?' We went back on air just a few minutes later and I recovered and could talk fine as more guests came on. I think that was the part that left some people in the room so confused. During the seizure, I couldn't put words together that were the least bit intelligible, but there was no other indication to anyone that I was having an epileptic 'aura', apart from those few who knew I was a sufferer. Then, straight after, I started talking normally again, as if nothing had happened. For the rest of the show I was more relaxed, even though I felt a little uncomfortable about who was going to come up with what stories. At least I knew another episode was extremely unlikely to occur, as it was rare for me to have two seizures in the one day.

After the show, nothing was said. Everyone got together for tea and coffee and a snack and we were all talking about old times, but no one brought it up. Part of that might have been people being courteous, although I think mostly they would have been confused about what they saw; maybe they just thought this bloke has taken one bump too many. Most of the banter was about all the things I did that would have *really* embarrassed me if they'd been put on the show.

Of course, Jacqui knew what was going on and it was heartbreaking for her. When it happened, she was behind the wall off-stage waiting to come on and knew straight away I was having a seizure. She said she felt like going out to see if everything was okay.

I was naturally very apprehensive after the program had finished. I thought, 'Will they show that part on the show or what?' Is *This Is Your Life* going to turn into a *60 Minutes* segment? I didn't know what to do. Even though I was working at Channel 9, I thought that if I started asking about the reaction to my 'turn', that might only set the ball rolling with interest from the news or current affairs people, who'd start questioning me about it. But if I said nothing, what had happened might leak out and I might be compromised into revealing the incident. I do remember walking out after the show had finished and going back to the newsroom, thinking, 'Oh well, I've got to cover the footy this afternoon, so life has to go on.' I looked at the boss, Lee Anderson, wondering what might be said and he just uttered something like, 'What have you been up to?' I wasn't sure if that was a veiled inquiry about what had happened or if I was being paranoid; I think he either didn't see it or hadn't been told at that stage.

I didn't know if the silence was good or bad but I decided I wasn't going to bring the subject up, and if it wasn't being mentioned to me, I'd let it go. I had no memory of what happened and I was pretty anxious when

I watched the show when it was televised a few months later. Fortunately, the big blooper was edited out and nothing was ever said about it; well, directly to me, anyway — I'm sure there was a fair bit of gossip through footy circles and the television industry.

It wasn't until I did an interview with Channel 9 in February 2008, a year after my surgery, that I saw the embarrassing footage. It was ironic that Mike Munro had been the *This Is Your Life* host; he was also the reporter when I was on *60 Minutes* years earlier talking about Jamie-Lee's cochlear implant, and I thought he hammered me a bit when a deaf do-gooder was flying off about us allowing Jamie-Lee to have the implant. Mike was great any other time I'd come across him and I quite liked the bloke.

I never stopped to think what might have happened to that pretty damning footage after that day I stuffed up. I found out when *A Current Affair* did the item on me in '08 and asked whether they could run the footage. I thought, 'Why not?' and called Mike — who I think was actually in the process of leaving Channel 9 after a long time with the network — to tell him *ACA* had requested to use the footage: did he know where it could possibly be?

He said, 'Yeah, I've just heard from *ACA* too. Mate, I'll tell you something — ever since that time, I knew something was going on. I didn't know what it was, but you didn't look in good shape. That film has been locked away ever since, so it wouldn't fall into the wrong hands. I know where it is and probably one other bloke does too, but he's never been able to get his hands on it without me.'

I thought that was just sensational of him and I told him I was happy for it to be released for this particular interview. He said that was fine, but I was the only one who he'd release it for and if I wasn't comfortable with it, he'd find a way to ensure it wasn't found. I assured him I was fine with it but would send something through on Channel 9 letterhead just to confirm it was indeed me and not someone impersonating me, which we had a laugh about. I always regarded Mike as a real gentleman who I had plenty of respect for ... and my respect increased further after that phone call.

It's interesting that I found out while doing this book that the journalist Paul Kent, who all but confronted me about my 'health issues' around that time (we think it was 2002) has said he knew I had epilepsy. I suspect someone may have said to him after the recording, 'You should have seen Wally gibbering away. There must be something wrong; maybe he's had too many knocks to the head.' But for someone to suspect it was epilepsy, they could only have got it from a good source who knew the details of my condition, because people generally didn't correlate that sort of behaviour with epilepsy. So I believe he either got the information from someone quite close to me, or he was obviously working in the wrong profession and being underpaid.

It seems something snuck out from someone; and maybe what happened on *This Is Your Life* was the catalyst for it spreading further than I ever knew.

ANOTHER PERSPECTIVE

By Mike Munro, This Is Your Life *host*

It was a great 'gotcha' … Wally Lewis had no idea a large news promotion and camera shoot had been set up just for our surprise for *This Is Your Life*. The sting went perfectly when I stepped forward with the red book in hand and told Wally the show would unfold in the next few hours.

Yet none of us had any idea that we would actually witness, for the first time, 'The King' being vulnerable and powerless. And it was in front of a large gathering of family and friends as he suffered an epileptic seizure — smack bang in the middle of recording the program.

Not long before the show, someone had confided in me that Wally was suffering from epilepsy, believing I should be aware of it before I put him through the surprise of a *This Is Your Life* tribute. I then remembered the couple of times I'd seen Wal completely lose it while broadcasting his sports segment live on Nine News. One second he was lucid and in total control, the next he was like a little boy getting all his words jumbled and back to front, but still ploughing on hoping he'd make sense. Unfortunately he didn't. The excuses at the time were that Wally had been working too hard and was suffering from an extremely bad virus or flu. Hardly anyone knew the sad truth that those occurrences were due to his epilepsy. My 'tip-off' would prove invaluable.

I was delighted to be doing Wally's *This Is Your Life*, having maintained a friendship with him, Jacqui and the children since I did a story for *60 Minutes* in 1992, involving their beautiful daughter Jamie-Lee.

We were about halfway through recording *This Is Your Life* when the great Ella brothers — Mark, Glenn and Gary — sent a message to Wally, remembering when they all played together in the Australian Schoolboys rugby union team. At the end of that message, Wal had his hand covering his face and I tried to look relaxed as I asked if he was okay. It was the first indication of something being wrong when he groaned and shook his head; the audience thought he was just reacting to the funny quips from the Ella boys. We then cut to vision of an incident early in his football career in which he copped a gruesome elbow to his throat, crushing his larynx. As I asked him about the incident, I noticed his demeanour had dramatically changed. He started to ramble; desperately trying to steady himself, trying so hard to keep his words together. But he was all over the place and I felt so sorry for him.

To bide time, I made out Wally was being modest. 'You're just too modest, Wally, and we know you don't like talking about yourself or your career,' I said. I knew that if the whole pre-recording was stopped, it would have been blown out of all proportion and embarrassed his family. I later learned that some of his family, who were at the rear of the studio and hadn't come on stage yet, wanted the show stopped there and then.

Fortunately, we kept rolling until the next guests walked out — three of his greatest football mates, Mal Meninga, Gene Miles and Trevor Gillmeister. The timing was perfect for Wally, because it meant the three guests would do most of the talking, giving Wally time to recover and slowly emerge from his petit mal seizure.

He didn't utter one word as the former footballers all delivered their individual anecdotes about Wally as he just kept smiling. After the footballers left the stage we had to go for a commercial break, which gave Wally more time to recover. By the time we started rolling the next segment he was his old self, particularly because Jacqui was the next guest on stage and she stayed with him on the couch until the end of the show. Afterwards, excuses were made once again for Wally's weird behaviour as the show rolled on, and at the usual after-show party, nothing much was mentioned.

Over the next few weeks, I had a number of calls from various sports journalists who wanted to know exactly what happened during the recording of the show. I avoided them all, although I have to say that by then I was extremely worried about Wally's safety and that of anyone in his car while he was driving. I asked the producer, Andrew Rodgers, to ensure Wally's epileptic fit was never used and to have it locked away.

When the program went to air a couple of weeks later, his seizure was well and truly cut out of the tribute.

As a journalist I was torn between a personal friendship, not just with Wally, but the whole Lewis family, and the fact that when I was told just before the show about his epilepsy, I was sworn to secrecy. I elected to say nothing; but as a friend I wanted to advise him to get help and that, in doing so, he would help so many others who suffer this condition.

Now that he's gone public with his condition, all these years later, he has become a real beacon of hope for thousands of epileptics around the nation.

NINE

IN FRONT OF THE CAMERA

M Y television career began because I was virtually ordered to get on camera by Brisbane Broncos chief executive officer, my old team-mate John Ribot. He said it would be good career preparation for me — and an excellent gesture by the club to one of our sponsors, Channel 10 — if I did a regular report from training each week about the Broncos in our inaugural season, 1988.

I'd only been doing the weekly report on the Broncos for just a few weeks when I was asked whether I'd be prepared to present the sports news for TEN a couple of nights a week. They were the official Brisbane World Expo station and would present the news from the Expo site along the Brisbane River.

My 'training' on how to handle life relying on the auto-cue consisted of being given a practice run of about 10 sports stories, being advised I did well and, to my amazement, being told, 'We'll start you tomorrow night.' Great. Playing in front of 30,000 at Lang Park didn't bother me too much, nor did being interviewed on TV or even doing the interviewing. But reading the news in front of six to seven thousand onlookers jammed up against a glass barrier, some of them half tanked and throwing 'brown eyes' at me, was a different proposition. But that was my introduction to being a sports presenter.

I was absolutely petrified the first day I had the task, so the news producer came out and said, 'We've made sure these stories are pretty simple. You won't have any trouble getting through them; you'll be right. You're used to playing in front of huge crowds; this is no different.' Yeah, right.

I thought, 'Even if I play in front of 60,000 people I feel comfortable because I know I've had 20 years' training, whereas doing this … I've had about 20 minutes!' Somehow I got through the first night without incident and I went straight to the bar afterwards for a couple of stress-breaking beers. The fear factor never left my body from then; even when I felt quite comfortable reading the auto-cue and delivering the stories with the right pitch and pause and all the little things that you're coached on.

On one of those first nights, a few of the hard heads around the place, and a young sports reporter called Terry Kennedy who is now host of 2KY's *Big Sports Breakfast* in Sydney, decided to give me an initiation I wouldn't forget.

I saw them all laughing as I walked on the set, naturally as nervous as hell. I mouthed, 'What's so funny?' and 'TK' told me to look at the tennis story I was about to read. Well, they'd put every difficult foreign name they could find in the list of results I had to read ... Martina Navratilova, and new players to the scene like Andrei Cherkasov, Natasha Zvereva and Goran Ivanisevic.

I quickly repeated them over and over in the minute or so I had before I had to start talking live to the camera, but I couldn't get Ivanisevic right even once. But when I was 'on' I somehow got it out correctly and was real proud of myself — all while the practical jokers were laughing and clapping off camera. In the next ad break, I called out, 'You bastards, I didn't think I would get that Ivanisav ... Ivanash ... oh bugger it.' I just couldn't get it right again; although I learned to pretty soon afterwards. I had no choice.

Making a faux pas was always at the back of my mind, as it is with any news presenter. There are plenty of things that can go wrong when you're live to air — as I very quickly found out.

In those days the auto-cue was a bit of plastic on a roller that would be manually pulled down in front of the camera, where a strong light shone over it and it reflected off a mirror you'd read from. These days it's all digital and computer generated and just comes down naturally in front of the camera you're looking at.

The golden rule is to have a written copy of each story, one per page, in front of you as a back-up if something goes wrong; so if you've ever wondered why in this high-tech age presenters still shuffle a bunch of pages in front of them, that's why. It was drummed into me in those early days, 'Don't forget, when you get on there just read your story; take your time, reach down, grab the paper the script is on, and as you finish one story, bring the next one to the top of the pile … and never get them out of order.'

I'd been reading the sport for a good few weeks and was becoming quite confident; Expo had finished and we were back in the Channel 10 studio. This one evening I got to the third story — a live read, to be followed by another live read, then another.

I had just begun the story by saying, 'And in the Around Australia Car Rally currently underway …' All of a sudden, the script on the auto-cue machine started to shake; it had become stuck and the woman operating the machine was unsuccessfully trying to free it. Things like this occurred occasionally and the newsreaders were trained to simply look down at their scripts and, after a brief pause while locating the words they'd just said, deliver the remaining lines. I looked down and was alarmed to see the second story still in front of me; I hadn't disposed of the hard copies of the stories as I'd finished reading from the auto-cue.

I thought, 'I'm in deep shit here ... what do I do to get out of this?' I decided to keep going, thinking I'd remembered most of the story. And after a long, clumsy pause, I continued. 'And in the Around Australia Car Rally currently underway, there were some problems for drivers today with an accident ... two ... two ... 250 kilometres southwest of Perth.'

As I went to deliver the next line, 'Officials believe ...', I thought, 'You dickhead — 250 kilometres southwest of Perth is in the middle of the Indian Ocean.' I stumbled on, eventually finishing the story the best I could, before spluttering out, 'And that's today's sport.'

Immediately after, we went to a commercial break and I began to slump back into the seat. There were two people on set with me, news readers Rob Readings and Anna McMahon. Rob said, 'You know, mate, I've been in this industry about 25 years now and I've been pretty embarrassed at times. You shouldn't worry about things like that — we all make mistakes.' I felt a little relieved and appreciated the settling words of support. Then he started laughing and added, 'Sorry, I can't tell any more lies ... that was the worst stuff-up I've ever seen on TV.' Thanks a lot.

It rocked me. Here I was just a few weeks into the job and I've been told I'd broken the record for the worst stuff-up! I had a host of people ask me over the next day or two, 'What happened on the news? I thought it was a bit of concussion.' That's when I realised playing footy on the big stage was a lot easier, and you're left a whole lot less vulnerable, than reading the sport news live.

I read the sport a couple of nights a week while the other times it was done by David 'Dasher' Fordham, a real professional experienced hand, who a little later moved to Channel 7 in Sydney. My role at TEN continued while I was at the Broncos, until I went down to the Gold Coast in 1991 to play there. I hadn't been there long when I went into the sports presenting role at SeaFM, which was a lot of fun ... except for the early starts.

There were a few male morning hosts, including Dean Miller, during the three years I worked at SeaFM, and a female, Suki Mead, and apart from me doing the straight sports news presenting, we had a ball ribbing each other. I said to them from the start that people wouldn't want me to talk just rugby league, so often I'd make the 'report' on the Seagulls very informal, but diplomatic, although one of the hosts would often start with, 'You can tell the Seagulls were beaten yesterday with how cranky Wally is this morning.'

When I returned to Brisbane in 1994, I began working for Channel 7. I'd been associated with Seven for a little while by being part of the Sunday morning *Sportsworld* program, filmed in their Sydney studios, and when they heard I was heading back to Brisbane, the station approached me. It was a lot more Queensland-friendly than getting stuck into by Roy Masters and Graeme Hughes, who liked to create interstate debate on *Sportsworld*. Geez, they used to give it to me and Queensland some times, which I didn't take too well until I quickly learned that that was television, designed to create a reaction, and I started giving it back to them in spades.

I was with the Seven Network for six years, and became increasingly confident in front of the camera and out on the road doing reports on any sport I was asked to do, plus reading the sport two or three nights a week. David Fordham returned to Brisbane with Seven during that period and was a great mentor and mate, and one of the best TV professionals and another good mentor, Pat Welsh, was also at Seven at the time (and still is). So I was surrounded by a really good crew and really enjoyed working there.

Not long after I arrived at Seven, ironically the first person I was asked to interview was Wayne Bennett. I said, 'You're kidding — that's like interviewing a rock.' Benny was well known for giving little away to the media and teasing them as much as he could. Anyway, a week later I said, 'Fine, I'll do it, but it won't be the questions you blokes ask like, "Do you expect to win? Who is the bloke you have to target to beat the opposition?" etc. I want to talk to him on a different slant, give a bit of an insight into coaching the club and what goes on.'

So I went to Wayne and told him how I wanted to do it and he said, 'Just fire away and we'll see how it goes.' So I opened with, 'Wayne, the first time …' He interrupted, 'Stop, whoa, whoa.' I said, 'What have I done wrong here?' He replied, 'If you're a journalist and you're going to start the interview, you have to say, "Well, Wayne." You listen to any interview or any press conference and it always starts with, "Well, Wayne." I said, 'You're a dickhead!' and we both had a bit of a chuckle.

I asked the question again, and he started laughing. But we got down to a serious interview and I said something like, 'There's plenty we read in papers and see on TV about the blokes who are in the footy team, but quite often it's the blokes behind the scenes that you have to deal with most of all.' He paused for a second and said, 'Yeah, that's right.' So we spoke about the backroom boys on his coaching team and their contributions and gave a bit of an insight into what makes a successful team, coach and organisation. At the end of it, he said, 'That wasn't bad; there were some good questions there ... but that doesn't mean I like you or want to talk to you again as a reporter,' and gave that half-smile of his.

I did very few interviews with him after that, but over the years it was more a succession of group media conferences after training at Red Hill (the Broncos' training ground), as often he'd only be available after the Saturday morning final training session.

I should background how Wayne and I got off on the wrong foot many years earlier, and have never been on each other's Christmas card list, although I'd like to think there's a fair bit of mutual respect there. In 1979, when I was playing at Valleys, we beat Souths — coached by Wayne — 26–0 in the Brisbane grand final. As you do, we hit the grog afterwards and I was still standing in my jersey, shorts and socks at the bar, absolutely legless well into the night! I was 19 and a typical smart arse with a few beers in me.

Our captain–coach Ross Strudwick came up to me and suggested I should call Souths Leagues Club and give them a bit of curry. So I got on the phone, put on as formal a voice as I could muster and said, 'Hello, can I speak to Wayne Bennett, please?' I was told, 'I'm sorry but Mr Bennett is at a private function — who is speaking?' 'It's Senior Detective Sergeant Merv Hoppner here from the city CIB. I'm after Mr Bennett to discuss a fairly important police matter.' Wayne was in the police force at the time, as a fitness instructor at the academy. Glen Hoppner was a mate of mine from the surf club and his father Merv was a fairly senior police figure at the time.

After a while, a voice came to the phone and fairly gruffly said hello. I said real smugly, 'Benny, how you going?' 'Who's that?' he asked. 'It's Wally Lewis from the Valleys club. Now when we walked off the ground today, it was 26–0, and when we left the ground an hour and a half later it was still 26–0. I'm just wondering whether you blokes have managed to score yet.'

The phone went *clunk*.

I put it to Benny years later that I realised it wasn't something I should have done and wasn't proud of, but I was drunk and put up to it by someone else. He said it wasn't him on the receiving end; he didn't take a phone call that night. I said, 'Well, if it wasn't you, it sure did sound like you.' Who's to know who was at the end of the phone, but it was a good gee-up, if not pretty bloody cheeky.

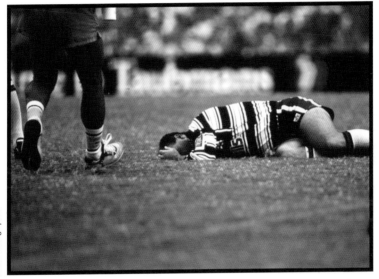

Concussion was suspected to have played a role in me developing epilepsy. Here I am snoring after a severe head knock, playing for Gold Coast against the Broncos at Lang Park (Suncorp Stadium) in 1992. The most embarrassing moment of my football career came when I left the field.

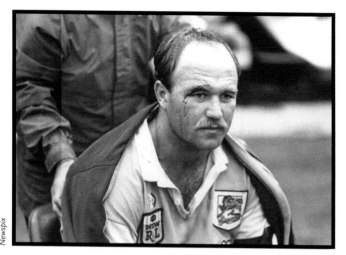

1990 was without doubt the toughest of my playing career. After being shifted to lock I broke an arm against St George. It effectively stopped me setting plenty of new records in the game.

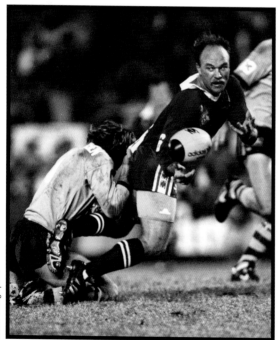

Playing in a State of Origin game was the ultimate challenge in rugby league and an opportunity to take part in one of the most intriguing sporting contests around the world that I never wanted to miss.

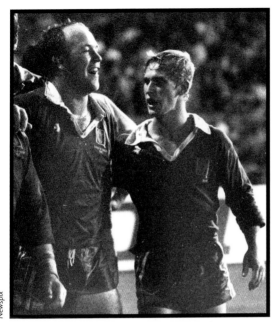

Staring down the barrel of three straight years of State of Origin losses, Queensland came from 1–nil down to draw the 1987 series (we won game three in Brisbane). Allan Langer and I sure did celebrate that night. He became one of the first to know I suffered epilepsy, although that wasn't by choice.

After exhaustive tests revealed that Jamie-Lee was profoundly deaf, I announced my retirement from representative football the following day after the final State of Origin game in 1991. Mitchell and Lincoln joined me in a lap of Lang Park, where I thanked the fans for the role they'd played in Queensland's success.

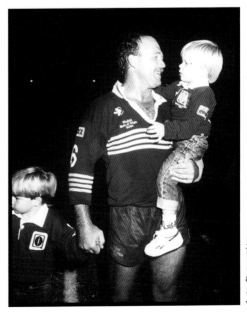

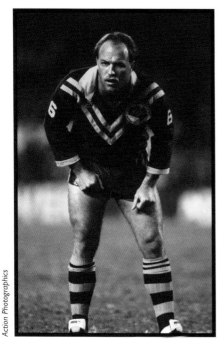

This shot was taken in the Test match against New Zealand at Lang Park in 1987, not long after I'd taken a head knock. It was a significant night – not only did we lose in one of the biggest Test upsets, during the resulting visit to hospital I was told I was an epileptic.

The Maroons created the greatest upset in Origin history to win the 1995 series 3–0. I'm hugging coach Paul 'Fatty' Vautin, while the blood pressure in team manager Chris 'Choppy' Close's face is about to increase his permanent tinge of red even further! Fatty was one of the few I told that I had epilepsy and we've been through a lot together over the years.

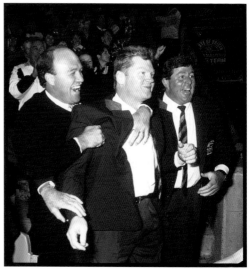

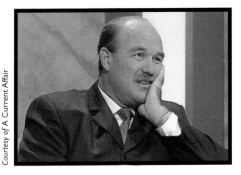

Courtesy of A Current Affair

Oh no. After being asked a question by host Mike Munro on *This Is Your Life*, I had a seizure and struggled to put words together, in front of an audience of family and friends, as well as the TV cameras.

It was a great surprise to see three of my favourite team-mates Mal Meninga, Gene Miles and Trevor Gillmeister at the *This Is Your Life* ceremony … but a bigger shock had just hit me: I was coming out of an epileptic seizure.

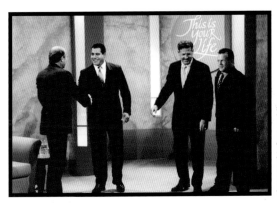

Courtesy of A Current Affair

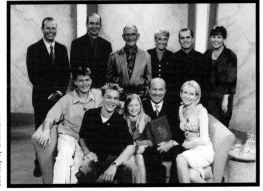

Courtesy of Channel 9

By the end of the show I'd recovered enough to smile, and had the support of my family. Top row (from left): brothers Heath, Scott, my father Jim, mother June, brother Eddie, sister Jean. Bottom row: Mitchell, Lincoln, Jamie-Lee and Jacqueline.

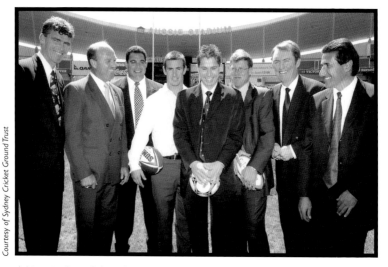

A historic shot of those lucky enough to captain an Australian sporting team at the Sydney Football Stadium. From left: Alex Tobin, me, Mal Meninga, Andrew Johns, Frank Farina, Nick Farr-Jones, Paul Wade, and Charlie Yankos. I couldn't stop looking at the post-op condition of Paul Wade's right temple and when I heard his slow speech that day, I swore I'd never have similar surgery.

An almost daily scene – on the Channel 9 news set with Bruce Paige and Heather Foord. It was usually an enjoyable experience as we swapped banter off-screen, but eventually it became an exercise of 'walking the plank' for me.

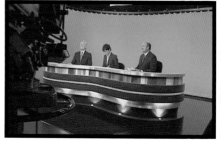

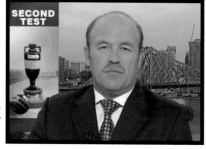

It turned out to be the most appropriately titled story of all. I was set to present the report of the second Test in the Ashes cricket series but it was me who failed to get off the mark when I couldn't utter the right words. It was the second 'Test' that I failed in November 2006; a second seizure in front of the camera within weeks.

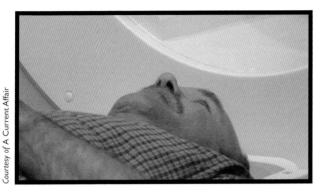

I'd had plenty of scans before, but this one at the Austin Medical Centre in Melbourne would decide my future. Assessing the position of the area causing my seizures would determine the possibility of surgery.

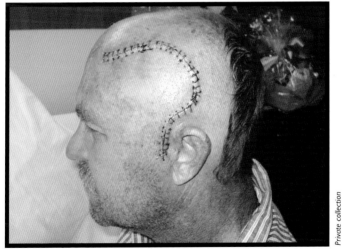

The shape of the incision may have been a question mark but there was no question I'd made the right move by having brain surgery – although it wasn't that clear in the first couple of months of my recovery period.

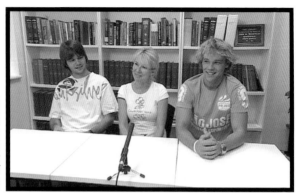

The relief in their faces was obvious as Mitchell, Jacqueline and Lincoln did a media conference after receiving a thumbs-up report on the operation from surgeon Professor Gavin Fabinyi.

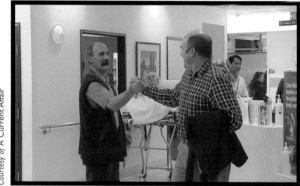

Upon returning to the hospital at the 12-month mark, I made sure I caught up with Les, the wardsman whose sense of humour helped relieve plenty of pressure for me inside the hospital.

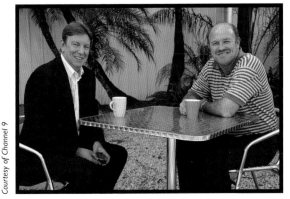

Courtesy of Channel 9

My Channel 9 workmate Lane Calcutt and I having a coffee in Melbourne a day or two before surgery. He knew I was 'back' when the light-hearted insults returned to our daily conversation once I was at work again.

Just over a week after the operation, a visit to Melbourne Storm training and a photo with Queenslanders Cooper Cronk, Dallas Johnson, Cameron Smith, Michael Crocker and Billy Slater helped break the boredom – although a similar shot appearing in the newspapers didn't impress me.

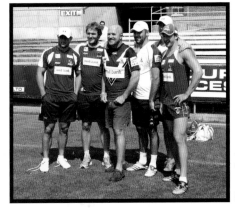

Private collection

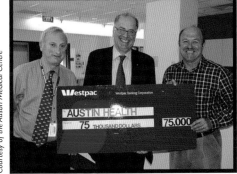

Courtesy of the Austin Medical Centre

A small way to say thank you to Professor Gavin Fabinyi and Professor Sam Berkovic – the two men who changed the course of my life – was to present them with a cheque for the proceeds of my TV and magazine interviews.

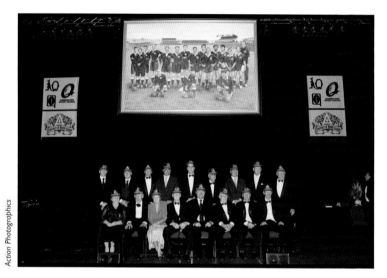

A great honour – being chosen in the Queensland Team of the Century.
There was only one thing that didn't fit during the photo session – the caps!

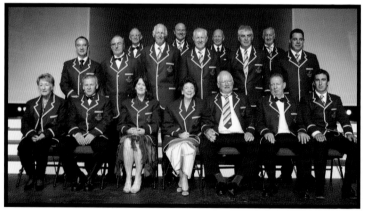

Being named five-eighth in the Australian Team of the Century was a truly
stunning recognition. But that night, the company of the men who'd created the
legend of the game in the decades before was even more priceless for me.

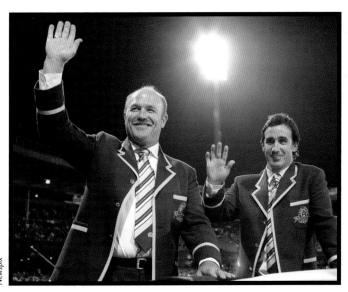

Andrew Johns and I during the lap of honour for the Team of the Century before the Centenary Test was played at the Sydney Cricket Ground in May 2008. I received a warm welcome from the crowd that I'd never experienced in Sydney before; it was very much appreciated.

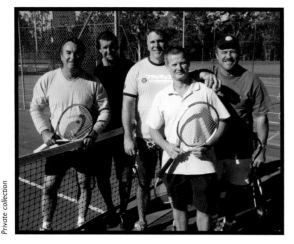

Private collection

It's a long way from Wimbledon! Best mates Mark Wilson, Allan Mohle, Peter Gamble and Brian Ball pose for the camera after another of our weekly epic battles.

I'd admired his achievements as captain of the Wallabies, but the life skills of my Channel 9 sports boss Andrew Slack are something very few people are blessed with.

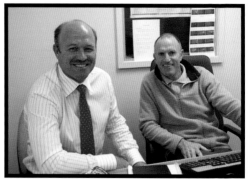

Courtesy of Channel 9

Yes, it's the real thing! At the Jack Newton Celebrity Golf Classic, I had an opportunity to meet the bloke I adored as a young music fan, Australian music legend Russell Morris. We also love short haircuts!

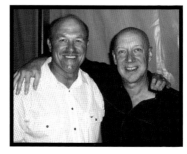

Private collection

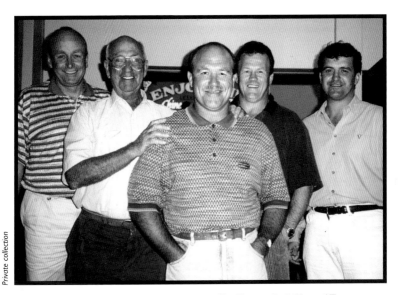

The 'Feedbag Club'. Once every month or so, Ken Brown, Dick 'Tosser' Turner,
Trevor Gillmeister, Greg Conescu and I used to dine together with our families.

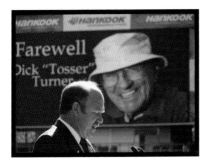

Farewelling former Queensland State
of Origin manager Dick Turner was one
of the saddest moments of my life. He
provided great support over the years.

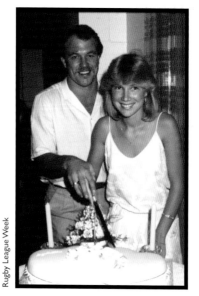

Rugby League Week

The first big step ... getting officially
engaged to Jacqueline Green in 1984.

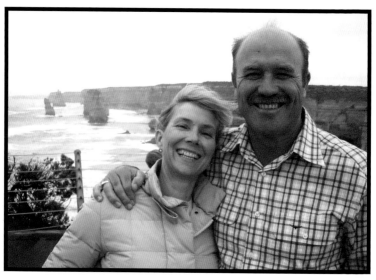

Private collection

The Great Ocean Road may be one of Australia's greatest tourist destinations,
but it also became a place that eased tension prior to surgery in February 2007.

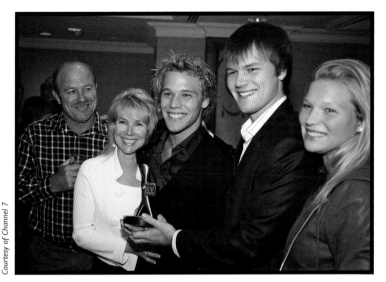

After watching the 2008 Logie awards in a Melbourne hotel room, the family raced across town to congratulate Lincoln for winning the 'Best New Talent' category. We were all very proud!

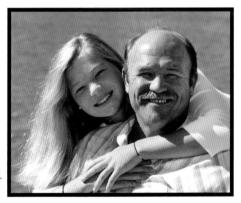

Our beautiful daughter Jamie-Lee. Her mother, brothers and I are very proud of her achievements, as she has never let her profound deafness stand in the way of anything.

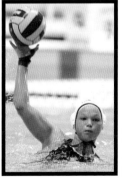

Some of the skills that have made her an Australian water polo representative.

Courtesy of Channel 7

Newspix

Private collection

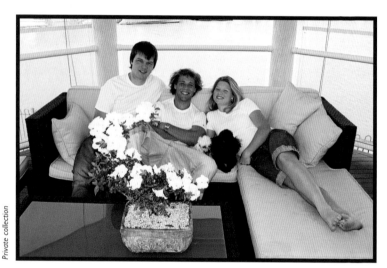

The trio who made my recovery so much easier. Mitch, Lincoln and Jamie-Lee out the back with our two mutts, Princess and Bronson.

I switched to the Wynnum club in 1984 and we belted Souths again in the grand final, 42–8. The next year I was given a job at the Queensland Rugby League as 'schools liaison officer' and by that time Wayne was the QRL coaching director. So we had to work in the same offices. I had to walk past Wayne's office to get to mine, and each morning we'd greet each other with 'Morning,' 'Morning,' and as I left, 'Afternoon,' 'Afternoon,' and not much else was ever said. One day, in 1986, Benny came into the office and said, 'Listen, we don't see eye to eye — you know that and I know that — but we have to start liking each other because I've just been appointed coach of the Queensland team.'

The fact was that we hardly knew each other really, and neither of us was the type of bloke who'd want to make the first move to rectify that. But I knew he was a damn good coach and when I was asked by Ron McAuliffe, the chairman of the Queensland Rugby League, who we should appoint as Queensland coach that year, I said there was only one bloke — Wayne Bennett.

We'd lost 2–1 in 1985. Des Morris was the coach, but being the first time we'd been beaten in five Origin series until then, the Queensland Rugby League decided a change in coach was necessary. Some people thought I had a role in instigating Des' downfall, because I'd had a run-in with him at the end of that season at Wynnum Manly where he was coach and I was captain, but that wasn't the case. By the time I was consulted, the decision had been made to find a new coach.

The Wynnum saga came about when I was asked to take some issues to him from senior players after we'd been beaten in the grand final. Somehow I was talked into going around to Des' place, hoping we could sort the problems out, but I also told him some players had even asked me to take over as captain–coach. He saw red then, accusing me of wanting his job and he ended up standing down. I reluctantly took over but the club was split in two over the whole ordeal. We ended up winning the competition and were a chance of securing back-to-back titles until it was announced that the club was broke. They'd indicated to players that a financial plan that was underway the previous season had collapsed. Players were in a state of financial disaster, some not being paid for three or four years. More bank loans were sought by players, but the rate of 18.9 per cent meant worse news was to come. The financial pressures even cost one player his life — tragically, he committed suicide.

We went down 3–0 in our first series under Wayne in 1986 — the first time any state had had a clean sweep — and at the end of the season he left the QRL for Canberra where he became co-coach with Don Furner, my Kangaroo coach in England that year. But there was little in any of the three Origin games in '86, which NSW won 22–16, 24–20 and 18–16. By Wayne's third season, we turned the tables completely for a 3–0 series win (after winning 2–1 in 1987) and no one had any doubts about his ability at that level. I enjoyed playing Origin under him as Queensland captain; I thought we combined well, and by that time he was Broncos coach and I was captain too.

I saw a lot of Broncos training during my time with Channel 7 — between 1994 and '99 — and enjoyed reporting on other sports and reading the sports news some nights. By that stage, I'd settled on the fact that television would, hopefully, be my career. I really enjoyed the job … but it got soured towards the end when the boss at Seven, Les Riley, came up with the idea that he didn't know how long rugby league would be the main interest in Brisbane given the success of the Brisbane Lions, who'd made the Australian Football League finals in 1997 in the first year of the merger between the Fitzroy Lions and Brisbane Bears.

When I questioned his wisdom, he told me that Channel 7 had a big investment in the telecast rights of the AFL and he wanted to send me to do the AFL games each weekend as a sideline comments man with former Aussie Rules legend Robert 'Dipper' Dipierdomenico.

I couldn't believe it. I said, 'What the hell? You want me to promote AFL? No way, I'm not doing it.' He told me I had no choice; that there was growing public interest in it, it was Seven's nominated sport and if people in Queensland knew that a league person like me was on the commentary team, it would be worth having a watch.

Despite my obvious reluctance, that's what I was ordered to do — even though I had no interest and very little knowledge about AFL. Dipper was great to work with: we'd have a chat early in the game, and again at quarter, half and three-quarter time, and he'd feed me a few lines of interest on what to talk about. Generally, I'd look at the game and tactics from a rugby league point of view and talk about how the games were similar or different, and ask the reason behind certain tactics that were used. I wasn't required for the full-time wrap-up; that was better left in the hands of those who knew what they were talking about. After a while, I'd shoot through after three-quarter time. That came about when I said to Dipper one day, 'Mate, I don't like to be rude, but I can't watch this any longer,' and I hopped in the car and drove home. That remained my routine from then on.

I covered the first few rounds of the following season, but I just couldn't keep up the charade. My contract had expired and I'd been onto the boss about getting a new one done, but he kept putting me off with, 'Yeah, it's coming, it'll be right.' I had the shits and in the end said I wasn't going to keep turning up to work without a contract. Just at that time, I heard through a third party that Channel 9 were interested in talking to me and wanted to know if I'd have time for a chat. I certainly would, and pretty quickly I signed a deal which involved doing sports news reporting and also doing sideline commentary on rugby league broadcasts. I only covered the games for one season, I think, and did more and more news and eventually began reading the sport as well, but I had no regrets about changing channels.

My seizures started to become more frequent, though, and the possibility that I'd have one on screen began to worry me. I was also working for Fox Sports, who covered all the NRL games except the two covered by Channel 9. That involved a lot of interstate travel doing two games a weekend, almost always with good mate and great commentator John McCoy and my old Test team-mate and Origin opponent Brett Kenny. Going to Perth and getting the 'red-eye express' plane back (departing around midnight), then going to another game the next day, was always the most harrowing, as I feared lack of sleep was the most likely trigger of a seizure.

We also did all the home games of the North Queensland Cowboys in Townsville; always an enjoyable trip with 'Macca' and 'Bert', which involved lunch in town at Sizzler and a heap of laughs on a Saturday, before we went out to the stadium to prepare for the 7.30pm kick-off. But what wasn't as enjoyable was that I could almost guarantee I'd have a seizure during that weekend.

Whether it was the heat that contributed, I'm not sure. It could sure be hot up there, especially if we were doing a day match. I remember one time telecasting The Super League World Nines, from the commentary box which wasn't air conditioned, and it was so unbearably hot in the box that John McCoy, Gary Freeman and I were sitting there with just our underpants on. A young lady was responsible for bringing drinks into the box, but after the shock of seeing us half naked, understandably she handed the task over to a young man.

I'd always try to get two or three hours' sleep in between lunch and when we had to go out to the stadium, and I'm sure that helped; but not enough at times. On several occasions, I had a seizure during the match commentary. I'd feel it coming on and sometimes I'd take my headphones off as a gesture to Macca not to cross to me. I'd put them down softly so the sound couldn't be heard over the air, John would give me the nod, then I'd grab my bottle of water and just sit there and look out until the seizure had passed. He said to me once, after this happened a couple of times, 'You just seemed to be off the radar a little bit.' He didn't understand why and thankfully didn't come back to me for an explanation.

Macca has only recently told me of a time when we were down on the sideline doing the match preview. He went to hand over to me for comment but said I seemed to be on another planet and I stumbled and stuttered at first, then started to look a bit blank; so he just took over himself. Apparently, there were some kids giving it to me over the fence with, 'What's wrong, Lewis?' I can't even remember it, as is the case with some other episodes.

I used to find the vast majority of the turns that I had happened because I was tired; then I'd have some sleep and feel a lot better. I always tried to target eight hours' sleep, and I'd certainly feel better for it.

From about 2000 onwards, I suppose I'd have an episode at least every three days although the frequency always used to vary. Half of them would last probably 90 seconds to two minutes, but some were four to five minutes before I was able to speak correctly without mixing things up and making a goose of myself.

It was only natural my performance on air with Fox Sports started to waver a bit, and became a bit inconsistent. I'd lost confidence and the worry of what might happen started to rattle me. But I thought that if I just took some 'time out' if I was hit by a turn during a game, I'd be okay once I got back into the swing of things. Maybe in hindsight, I should have told my employers about my condition — but I just wanted to keep it to myself as long as I could.

After the 2003 season, my seventh with Fox Sports, I hadn't heard whether I was on the commentary team for the next season. They just didn't get back in contact with me, so I rang the boss at the start of the following year and said, 'I was just wondering whether I've got the bullet; I haven't heard from anyone.' I got the old 'I'm not sure what's going on yet — we'll get back to you'. After a few more weeks of silence I told him, 'Mate, if I'm getting the flick, just let me know.' I was wondering whether someone had let the cat out of the bag about my epilepsy, but I don't think that was the case. In the end, I was given the boot from the match commentary but was kept on for a couple of years doing the midweek show, *NRL on Fox*. I've heard since that they thought I was better suited to that and had lost my edge a bit as a co-commentator.

At Channel 9, after some close calls, I was in constant fear that I'd have an on-air seizure. In the end, it was like putting my career at risk every night, and being subject to devastating embarrassment, if I 'lost it' in front of the camera. On a couple of occasions I'd been only minutes away from getting the make-up on ready to do the news, thinking, 'Here we go spinning the gun barrel again … is the bullet going to go off tonight?'

By that stage I was taking close to the maximum dosage of Tegretol, Dilantin, Topomax and Keppra. I couldn't have been loaded up with more medication; the only alternative was major surgery — and I wanted to avoid that.

The frequency of the seizures, what time of day they would occur and how bad they would be was a lottery. I might go for a week or 10 days without one but once it reached 10 days, and often I'd think that was because I'd had a pile of sleep and rest, I knew one was coming for sure. I could get one every three or four days, sometimes just mild ones; then for no apparent reason I'd get one in the morning, one in the afternoon and then one next morning — three in 24 hours. Having said that, it was rare to have more than one on the same day. I used to be so relieved if I had one early in the day; I'd think, 'Thank Christ, I've had that one, I'll be okay to do the news tonight.'

When I felt one coming on at work, the challenge was to get out of view of everyone else and get to the toilet before it was in full force. So I found a back-door route to the dunny, which meant I wouldn't have to go past Andrew Slack's office, and I'd have my routine of ensuring my mobile phone was at my ear, so people would think I was talking and wouldn't try to get my attention.

I used to walk past an area where old tapes are kept, past the librarians' room, down a set of stairs, into where the kitchen is — and it would usually be empty — leave the building, go towards the car park, come back into the building via another entrance, into the dressing room … to my isolated haven, the toilet. If Slacky wasn't in his room, I'd take the short cut past his office which would save me 50 metres. I don't know what I looked like while I was walking on my little course, whether there seemed any irregularity to other people, but I sure wasn't going to slow down to find out.

I'd guess I did that 20 times over four or five years. The first thing I'd do was to drop my strides and sit on the toilet so I wouldn't piss my pants. I'd stay there for seven or eight minutes until I knew it had passed and I was okay; that I was fully 'with it' again. Inevitably, when I wandered back someone would say, 'C'mon, where's the stuff you have to work out before going on air?' Or 'Where have you been? I have to give you this.' I'd act calm and say everything was fine, and that I had another 15 or 20 minutes before I had to get ready.

A lot of the time I'd actually have the seizure while I was walking to the toilet. My biggest fears were either that I'd start pissing myself or that I'd have to respond to someone who wanted to talk to me. So, pretending I was talking on the mobile phone would be a successful diversion. Sometimes if I was sitting at my desk and felt one come and couldn't get out of sight, I'd reach for my phone to distract others from talking to me and sit there until it had passed.

Naturally, the worst situation was if I had gone through make-up and was either at the sports desk ready to go with the news, or just about to sit down at the news desk — that was the point of no return.

One time I was about to read the news and I had the countdown from the commercial break; I remember hearing '90 seconds' as that dreaded feeling hit my body again. I was thinking, 'Oh shit,' and went white as a ghost. Heather Foord kept saying, 'What's wrong, Wal, what's wrong?' I didn't know what to say, and probably more importantly I couldn't put the words together to answer her. I kept looking at her. I can still remember hearing '10 seconds', and then …

I looked down and started reading the first paragraph. It was something like: 'The … the … Aust- … ralian … c- … cricket t-t-t- … team have won … this afternoon's battle with New Zealand (by this stage I was starting to get it together) … after skipper Ricky Ponting chalked up an unbeaten 104 at the MCG.'

Fortunately, it had been one of the briefer seizures, which lasted maybe 45 or 50 seconds. We went to the vision and I said to Heather and Bruce Foord something like, 'Could I have screwed it up any worse than that … gibber, gibber, gibber!' They just laughed but had no idea how big a bullet I'd just dodged. By the time the camera was back on me, I wasn't too bad and read the rest of the sports news fine.

Another time, I was walking down to the newsroom as I started to have a turn, and I just hoped it'd be out of the system by the time I reached there. I don't recall what was going on or if anyone said anything to me; I would have pretended I was reading my notes. Fortunately, it was a minor seizure and had passed just in time for me to hear the start of the countdown.

The nerves would always settle after the first story: if I got that out, I used to think, 'That's not too bad; I'm in the clear.' I asked the doctor later whether fear or anxiety or pressure had anything to do with bringing a seizure on, because I had three or four when I'd just started, or was about to start, the countdown. Not once did it happen during the second or third story. He admitted pressure had something to do with it, and maybe the build-up before the first story might have made me more intense, and after that I'd relax my body.

Ask anyone who suffers epilepsy; once you've had a seizure, you're exhausted afterwards. So it was a big enough concern if I had one in the afternoon, more so than just before the news. I'd try to get away for even half an hour and close my eyes for a while. I was worried about getting through the remainder of the day without the rest that my body was crying out for. I would crash on the lounge when I got home from work each night and wouldn't be much of a source of conversation; invariably I'd fall asleep in front of the television set.

But the biggest fear I had was whether anyone had seen me or knew about my behaviour, and whether I'd have to cough up an explanation. I'd always try to regularly save whatever was on my computer screen too, so I wouldn't lose it if I had a turn during the day.

However, that didn't always go according to plan, because of terrible lapses in my memory. My short-term memory loss — forgetting what I was doing or told just minutes earlier — was frustrating and rather scary. Eventually, when I went for the scans before my operation, it was confirmed that my memory had been drastically damaged by the epilepsy, which was no surprise to me.

On a number of occasions while working at Channel 9, I'd ask Andrew Slack if there was a story he wanted covered. Usually Slacky would reply with something like,

'Yeah, we'll get you to do a story on the footy. Just see what comes out of today's training session, and if there's something to come from Sydney later, you might be able to add that.' I could normally handle those requests quite comfortably, especially considering there was only one story base: rugby league. But several times a simple job list would prove to be a real hurdle. Slacky might say, 'We'll get you to do a package. Start off with the Queensland cricket training session with a grab from one of the players about how they'll go this weekend, then cut to the surfing titles in Hawaii and get a few good shots in; then finish with the golf tournament underway in the USA. And make it about one minute all-up. So it's cricket, surfing and golf.'

There'd be another 10 or 15 seconds of general conversation between us before I'd leave the room to walk back into my office 10 metres away. I'd sit down and prepare to get started by typing the story list into the computer to search for vision and 'wire' copy. It should have been something simple like typing 'cricket/surfing/golf' and then I'd type '1.00' into the time slot. Occasionally, by the time I sat down at my desk I'd forgotten what Slacky had just asked me to do. I'd sit for a couple of minutes, hoping it would come back to me and I'd look at the stories locked into Channel 9's Sydney and Melbourne studios, hoping that would prompt me.

Sometimes it helped, but many times it didn't, and I'd walk sheepishly back into Slacky's office and ask again what he'd just asked me to do. It mightn't have worried the respected former Australian rugby union captain too much, but I wasn't exactly giving the common sense image of rugby league players much of a boost.

Also, when I started to construct the stories I'd have long pauses while writing scripts, trying to think of the most obvious word that I needed. I'd get frustrated and ask for someone else's input and they'd invariably laugh and say it was a legacy of getting old; but I knew it was more than that in my case. I attempted to overcome it by buying a thesaurus that would provide alternate words, and that came in handy — most of the time.

There were occasions when I'd completed my script, including quotes from sportspeople, and had it all ready to cut the story, but then I'd feel a seizure coming on. I'd sit quietly and ride it out and would only come back into the real world several minutes later when the phone rang or somebody entered the room. It might have been Andrew or news director Ron Kruger asking where the script was. I'd go to the computer to call it up but couldn't find it; it wasn't in the list of news stories logged into the system, nor could I see it in my personal files. I'd assume that I didn't save the story or had clicked the wrong button on the computer while attempting to save it during the 'turn' and had inadvertently deleted it.

I'd be left totally confused and exasperated by what I must have done. Imagine being at the end of the day all ready to put the items together for the sports news and … one is missing; gone out of the system. I, or someone else, would have to start all over again. On a couple of occasions, there was only 10 or 20 minutes before the item was required ready to go to air, which left no time to re-create it properly. They'd have to grab some footage and put down a very basic summary of events, patched up very poorly, to cover my arse, or lift the item from Sydney or Melbourne and run it exactly as they had. It ensured the trip home wasn't one to enjoy, I tell you; I'd be very down on myself, often wondering how long those stuff-ups could continue before I was called in to be told that sort of performance could no longer be tolerated.

I was living a terrible lie and taking a terrible chance with my television career. It was affecting my daily demeanour, my self-confidence and self-esteem and, looking back now, I was kidding myself thinking I could live my life like that for much longer.

Eventually I had to come clean, and I spilled everything to Andrew Slack — fearing all along I might be talking myself out of the television industry. What I found instead was amazing support and compassion from some great people at Channel 9 — for which I am eternally grateful. In fact, Slacky got me out of the shit right at the death a couple of times. As I'll explain later, it was lucky he always had a coat and tie on the back of his office door!

ANOTHER PERSPECTIVE

By John McCoy, former Fox Sports colleague

I CONSIDER myself extremely fortunate to have been a rugby league caller in Brisbane during what was a golden era for the game in Queensland. There were so many outstanding players — the likes of Mal Meninga, Gene Miles, Greg Dowling, Bob Lindner and Dale Shearer — who formed the backbone of the Queensland State of Origin and the Australian Test teams.

As outstanding as those players were, Wally Lewis was simply in a class of his own. However, when I look back on Wally's career, the fondest memories were of his formative days in the late-'70s/early-'80s at Valleys. Here was this young kid with unbelievable talent and, to his credit, coach Ross Strudwick gave Wally a licence to show those skills.

As a commentator, I always had a very good rapport and working relationship with Wally. Our paths would cross frequently away from the football field at many sporting functions and award dinners where I'd be asked to interview him. We got to know each other pretty well and I'd like to think that the great respect I had for Wally was mutual.

Later, we worked together in television commentary for Fox Sports; often along with a third member, Brett Kenny, on the sideline. It was fascinating to sit and listen to the two of them talk football, because personality-wise they are as different as chalk and cheese, yet are great mates. Wally has spoken of some of our trips away and the legendary lunches at Sizzler in Townsville, but they were so much fun for the simple reason that we all thoroughly enjoyed each other's company and that makes for an easy transition to the commentary duties.

It was the late Dick 'Tosser' Turner who first hinted to me that Wally may be epileptic. It was at a FOGS luncheon where I was the MC; I had a meeting with Tosser, the FOGS chairman, before the lunch began, and Wally's name came up. He told me of his fears that Wally may have a medical problem and that the symptoms were akin to epilepsy. I don't know whether Tosser had any actual medical basis for his comment or whether it was just a hunch from his vast experiences of life, but what he said struck a chord with me.

Sometimes Wally could become rather vague when in a discussion, seeming to drift off the track, then all of a sudden his train of thought would return and he'd continue as normal. That trait did sometimes bring forward comments from people that 'he's had too many hits to the head'. I knew that was certainly not the case. I've met enough former boxers who were, unfortunately, 'punch-drunk' to know that it was nothing like Wally's situation.

Should I and so many other of his close friends have tried to do something about it? That's a difficult question to answer, and even in hindsight I'm not sure that we could have helped. The reason being that Wally was given medical attention and it was thus a private matter. People like me with absolutely zero medical knowledge had no right to interfere or make uninformed suggestions. All we could do was help Wally if we were together and he began feeling unwell.

The turns that Wally took while reading the television news and at the taping of *This Is Your Life* are well documented, but he did have a similar problem at a Cowboys game in Townsville. I remember the flight from Brisbane to Townsville that morning because we'd only just taken off when Wally asked for a blanket. Now that in itself was probably not unusual as he'd often do so on an early-morning or late-night flight, but this was mid-morning on a sunny day with a pleasant cabin temperature. I asked if he was feeling okay and he said he was fine.

It may have had no bearing on what happened later, as at lunch he was his normal self and afterwards he had a rest as was always the case. He seemed fine on the way to Dairy Farmers Stadium and I can remember Brett, Wally and me being highly entertained by a colourful description on the local radio of a rugby league match from Cape York, where there were no modern innovations such as kicking tees, so the goal-kicker just picked up the nearest cow pat!

Wal was in good spirits until we went to the sideline during the reserve grade match and began recording the telecast opener, at which stage he became incoherent. We stopped the recording and even when I asked him if was feeling unwell, the question didn't register and he just looked at me vaguely, not knowing whether he was in Townsville or Cape York. Naturally, whenever Wally and Brett were near the sideline fence, the crowd would swell to hear what they had to say. I remember one fellow calling out in a loud voice, 'What's wrong, Wal, are ya pissed?' Now that is something that Wally Lewis could never be accused of.

The 'turn' that night in Townsville passed as quickly as it had arrived and by the time Brett and I had recorded the opener, Wal had recovered. As a precaution, we had Brett stay with us in the broadcast box rather than be on the sideline, but there was no further problem. Interestingly, I remember the drive back into Townsville after the game and we were still laughing about the Cape York call which Wal could remember clearly, but when the recording of the opener was mentioned he had little or no recollection.

One of Wally's most enduring traits is his generosity and patience with fans. It's only when you spend some time in his presence that you realise how demanding a task that can be. There is a constant stream of people wanting autographs and photos and never once have I seen Wally be anything but utterly co-operative. He knows full well that those people have given him the iconic status that he enjoys and the many material benefits that flow from such a position.

One weekend that best exemplifies his patience was when Fox Sports had us calling a Cowboys v Broncos match on Saturday night in Townsville and a Newcastle v Manly game in Newcastle on the Sunday. We arrived back at our Townsville units after the game and arranged to meet at 5am next morning to catch the flight to Brisbane.

I was first down to the foyer to be greeted by a fan in full Broncos outfit who'd found out where we were staying and had camped in the foyer all night to get Wally's autograph. When Wal came down a few moments later, I asked him for the keys to the car so I could pack our gear while he had a chat with the young fellow. Unfortunately, the car keys were missing and there was desperation as Wal flung open his bags and briefcase in a futile search, then told the bloke to wait while he went back to the room. Time was ticking away and we had to catch the plane or we wouldn't get to Newcastle.

The keys had disappeared and we frantically called a cab only to be told that as there was such a crowd in town from the Broncos match, there was a 90-minute wait. When the concierge told the cab company who the cab was for and the necessity to get to the airport, the cab was there in about two minutes flat. I still have visions of Wal posing for pictures as the cab was pulling away, and signing a jersey, flag and football through an open window as the fellow ran along beside. Incidentally, we made the plane as the doors were closing; the keys were never found.

When we reached Newcastle after a drive from Sydney, we were told the car park was full but the attendant did find us a space in the last row. That meant that after the game we had to be the last to leave and the word quickly spread among the Novocastrians that if you wanted Wally Lewis' autograph, here was your chance because the King had no escape route. Without exaggeration, the queue would have been at least 100 metres long and didn't seem to ever get shorter. Wally must have had writer's cramp by the end, but he signed every autograph, had a chat to each fan and posed for hundreds of photos.

Wally is extremely fortunate to have such a wonderful family and they have been a rock to him during his battle with epilepsy; but as Jacqui says, the ultimate reward for them is having the 'old Wally' back. Wally Lewis is without question one of the greatest athletes that our sports-loving nation has produced, but away from the spotlight there is a very genuine, generous bloke who has faced a major health crisis with an admitted fear and self-doubt that football followers never thought would be in his make-up.

However, once the decision to go ahead with the delicate operation was made, he produced those same qualities of grit, determination and will to win that we admired on football fields for so many years. Wally Lewis is a bloke who I am honoured and privileged to call a mate.

TEN

COMING CLEAN

I WAS walking down to the news reading, set to do what I must have done over a thousand times: presenting sport on the evening news half-hour. Then it hit, as usual with no warning … another bloody seizure. This time, it came at the most inconvenient time.

I knew it was going to be touch and go. I was hoping the seizure would pass in time for me to shake myself off before going in front of the camera; but it wasn't looking good.

I walked upstairs from make-up and past Slacky's office. I wasn't consciously looking for an escape route — I couldn't think about anything in those confusing moments when I was subject to a 'turn' — but I found one.

On my way back to my office, Slacky looked at me and asked if everything was alright. I don't know whether I just shook myself or tried to utter some sort of answer, but he didn't need one. He could see I definitely wasn't okay. He was the one man at my work who knew what was happening, and that quick decisive action was needed.

He stood up and reached behind his door to reveal a coat and tie sitting on a hook. Slacky is one of those solid, unflappable personalities you'd want by your side in a crisis; a thorough professional who'd weathered his own personal tragedies but showed enormous strength of character. And unlike me, he could put a tie on in perfect position without the use of a mirror.

Andrew threw on his coat, called the producer to advise that he'd be reading tonight's sport instead of me and to change the on-screen graphics, grabbed the scripts that were in my hand and, amazingly considering the circumstances, sat next to Heather Foord and Bruce Paige and gathered his thoughts quickly enough to look at the camera after hearing, 'And now with tonight's sport, Andrew Slack,' and do a thoroughly professional job in presenting the sports news.

That scenario happened twice in a space of a few months, both times between 6.05pm and 6.10pm. I'd dodged two more bullets, but it remained our secret.

I'd decided to confide in Slacky about my epilepsy in 2002 (I think); it had got to the stage where I thought I couldn't hide my dilemma from my immediate boss any longer. I walked into his office one morning and said I needed to talk to him. I offered, 'There are not a lot of blokes I trust in the world but you're one of them; mate, I've got something to tell you ...' Then I spilled out everything; how I'd increased the medication to try to nullify the seizures, which had no general pattern of frequency; how they affected me at work and how I'd had to adapt my lifestyle but had become less confident in public; what he should look for if I was having a 'turn' but, also, that so far I'd been able to just ride them out at work and by the evening I was usually fine.

He sat back and asked a question every now and then as I spoke for probably half an hour; then he asked if anyone else at the station knew. I assured him he was the first one, but I understood that he'd have to notify the station manager Lee Anderson, which he duly did. I later had a briefer discussion with Lee, who appreciated my frankness and sort of just said he was there to support me, and let's get on with business. It was support that I greatly appreciated.

From that day, I've been very fortunate to witness the compassion from people at Channel 9, from senior management right through to my work colleagues when all was revealed in late 2006. They have no idea how much that has meant to me and my family.

While the television industry is perceived as being extremely cut-throat, impersonal, fraught with petty jealousies and egos and about ratings and advertising income — particularly in harsh economic times — Nine have stuck by me beyond what they were required to. One insider at the station once told me that perhaps the station executives felt partially responsible for my situation due to the pressure being placed upon me working in such an industry. I countered it by saying that there's pressure in a lot of industries these days, not just the media, and no one but me is responsible for having fits.

Naturally I was concerned that, especially if there had to be a pruning of staff in tough times, my situation would make my position more vulnerable — but that was the risk I had to take. I had to come clean. And I felt relieved I had, even though I again didn't want it becoming common knowledge.

On both those occasions that Andrew Slack had to cover for me at the 11th hour, I was naturally embarrassed and apologetic, and each time I went to my doctor to inform him of what had happened and inquire about what more could be done. But, before my two on-air meltdowns in 2006, I had only a few close calls over eight years at Channel 9, plus my *This Is Your Life* episode, so maybe that's why I thought I could keep going as I was. Yet, in the back of my mind, the fear never subsided.

Slacky is a special bloke. A former Australian rugby union Test captain, his working career actually began as a teacher at Villanova College in Brisbane, the college he attended as a student. He is naturally a legend there and one of the ovals is named after him. He had an illustrious playing career that included 29 Tests for Australia as a clever centre, and he captained the Wallabies in 19 of them — including the historic Grand Slam tour of 1984 when the Australian team became the first to beat all five major European Nations (England, Scotland, Ireland, Wales and France). He also held the record for Queensland appearances with 133 before it was broken by Mark Connors in 2006. He joined Channel 9 in 1988 as sports director and he is very respected in the industry.

Only a few months after I confided in Slacky with my personal information, he called me into his office to take me into confidence about a big decision he was confronting — whether to accept an invitation to coach the Queensland Reds in the Super 12 competition. He'd been an Australian selector since 2000 but this was an opportunity to go full-time back into the sport. While I appreciated him asking for my thoughts, I said, 'Mate, if you're asking my opinion, I think you've already made up your mind.' I think he was just searching for confirmation he had made the right choice. I didn't want to put too much of my opinion forward as it had to be his decision entirely. I then honoured his wishes not to breathe a word to a soul until he'd announced his decision; I didn't even mention it to Jacqui.

Slacky resigned as sports director and coached the Reds for the 2003 season, but it didn't go as well as he would have liked and he was back at Nine by the end of the year. In the meantime, well-known Channel 9 sports reporter/presenter Chris 'Bomber' Bombolas (who incidentally went to the same schools as me at the same time, Cannon Hill State School and Brisbane State High) took over as sports director. Bomber went back to his previous role when Slacky returned, before eventually going into politics in 2006, winning the seat of Chatsworth for Labor. I decided not to tell Bomber about my epilepsy and just hoped for the best in Slacky's absence.

And I didn't notify anyone else in the ensuing years, even football mates and family friends, until the shit hit the fan and I had to make a public confession on the last day of November in 2006.

ELEVEN

THE LAST RESORT

I HAD done a complete about turn when it came to the
subject of brain surgery. From ruling it out of hand as
even the last resort, I'd quickly come to the realisation that
it was my best chance of ever having a 'normal' life again.
Suddenly, nothing was going to stop me from having the
delicate operation. I was desperate.

I haven't explained until now why I was so dead-set
against the surgery that has been a revolution to many
sufferers like me. Dr Noel Saines at the Wesley Hospital
had mentioned it to me probably some time just either
side of the new millennium, and I considered it for a while
as an option if medication failed to curb my seizures,
which were becoming more frequent.

Then one day in 2002 I was invited to go to the Sydney
Football Stadium, where all captains of Australian sporting
teams that played at the stadium were gathered to open a

'Captains Bar and Dining Room'. At the function were the likes of Mal Meninga, Andrew Johns, Charlie Yankos, Nick Farr-Jones and former Socceroos captain Paul Wade.

Paul, who captained the Australian soccer team 46 times, has a similar story about epilepsy to mine. He'd had auras for many years without knowing what they were and was diagnosed with epilepsy a couple of years before he retired in 1996. He worked as a commentator with Fox Sports and he, like me, suffered the ignominy of stuffing up live on air, prompting him to go public with his condition and also to have the brain surgery.

Wade had been interviewing Socceroo Paul Okon straight after an Australia–France game at the Melbourne Cricket Ground in 2001. During the interview he had a seizure, started stammering his words and lost control of his hand movements. Apparently he was 'offside' with a few of the players because of public criticism of their performances and Okon interpreted Paul's behaviour as taking the piss out of him.

Okon was obviously riled and as he walked away he gave Wade the 'finger', which was captured on television. The embarrassing situation caught on camera, like mine six years later, left Paul with no option but to come clean on what had happened. He later went in for similar surgery to mine, although I believe a different part of the brain was removed.

I knew nothing about any of his on-air drama at that stage and met Paul for the first time at the function at the SFS. We had to walk out to the centre of the playing field, with our suits on for a photograph, and I noticed Paul walking slowly and gingerly. I asked one of the other soccer guys what the problem with him was and was told that Paul was recovering from surgery; I thought back surgery or something like that. Then I noticed a lump almost the size of an egg on the right side of his forehead. I then asked what type of surgery and was told, 'Brain surgery for his epilepsy.'

That naturally grabbed my attention very quickly, so I turned around and went back to Paul and asked him how he was going. 'Yeeeeahhhhh … reeeeeally goooooood … nooooow, thaaaanks.' I said, 'How long ago did you have the operation?' I think he said nine or 10 months and that he'd been a real mess for a long time. Others then told me how terrific he was now and how well he was recovering!

I was stunned. That was the end of any chance that I was going to submit myself to brain surgery. I thought if that's the Holy Grail of surgery for epilepsy, you can shove it up your arse. I went back to Dr Saines a few days later and told him he could flick surgery from option number three right down the list until he'd run out of numbers. I said there was no way in the world I was going to feel like, or look like, Paul Wade did.

That attitude changed quite dramatically after my meltdown in front of the cameras and the start of the path that led me to the eminent professor Sam Berkovic. When I'd completed that quite emotional 'consultation' with Professor Peter Silburn on 7 December 2006 and he finished his summary with, 'Right, you're going to Melbourne; you're going to see Sam Berkovic,' I had complete trust in Professor Silburn's suggestion, even though I knew nothing of Professor Berkovic and far less than I thought I knew about epilepsy. Yet for the first time in a long while, I felt calm and relieved. It was the first step towards a new chapter in my life, but I felt it was a big step. When I got home I immediately jumped on the computer and 'Googled' the name Sam Berkovic, and the response left me more than happy with Professor Silburn's direction that I head to Melbourne.

A week later, Jacqui and I were at the Austin Medical Centre at Heidelberg. I'm rarely nervous when meeting people for the first time, but there was such an aura around this man I was in awe of, I was a bit jittery. During the several hours I spent searching the internet for information on Sam, I discovered that his achievements were stunning. I thought epilepsy involved 'petit mal' or 'grand mal' seizures, but I soon discovered epilepsy to be a far more complex problem, with 57 different forms of the disease. It was no surprise to see why Sam had been spoken of so highly, and was so highly respected worldwide; he had discovered 38 of the 57!

Professor Berkovic agreed that undergoing the PET scan was the best path to follow. He explained what the tests were targeting and asked our thoughts. I described how I felt my options had been reduced, and while I strongly favoured surgery, I agreed that all the alternatives should be placed on hold until information from the upcoming scans was produced.

I felt comfortable I was in good hands and I slept quite well on the return flight to Brisbane. When we arrived home it was a beautiful afternoon and after opening the back doors to let a nice breeze in, I stretched out on the lounge and began flicking through the television channels to see what was on. I was going through the Fox Sports channels when I came across a weekly soccer program. Just as I was about to switch to another channel, I was brought to my feet; I'd noticed a face that I remembered all too well. I screamed out to Jacqui, 'That's Paul Wade! That's Paul Wade! He's on television!' Jacqueline had no idea what I was talking about and asked what was wrong, but her last words were drowned out. 'That's Paul Wade …

"Wadey" … he's the one that …' I had such a big lump in my throat I couldn't finish the sentence.

I noticed the scar on the right side of Paul's head, but what stunned me more than anything was the speed of his discussion. As he described an insight into the game's tactics he was talking at the same speed as anyone else, far quicker than when I'd met him years earlier at the Sydney Football Stadium. He appeared to be back to his old self. I began to choke; I realised I had tears streaming down my face. The fear of surgery quickly disappeared. I thought, 'I've been dodging and weaving for years about having surgery based on what I observed of Paul Wade after his operation, and look at him now.' I felt so happy for him too.

That coincidence of seeing Paul Wade on television at that time wasn't lost on me; it was as if it was further confirmation that I was doing the right thing going down the path of surgery. I felt calm and quite content for the first time in a long while.

I must say it was one of the quietest Christmases I've had, spent on the Sunshine Coast. We'd made all the arrangements for the February trip back to Melbourne; finding a hotel near the hospital, booking flights and getting familiar with that part of the city. I'd agreed to do an interview with my old Channel 9 colleague Lane Calcutt, and when he arrived there was little of the bagging and counter-bagging sessions that had become common between us.

To be honest, I didn't really want to go ahead with the interview, but I thought I would just come clean and get it over and done with in the one interview on my own station, and that would hopefully be the end of it as far as a public explanation went. While Lane was very careful with his questions, I opened up and declared that I'd had a gutful of battling unsuccessfully with the disease. When he asked if surgery could now be an option, I replied, 'I'll do whatever it takes to get rid of it. I don't want to battle it any more because I'm sick and tired of being sick and tired.'

There was a lot of media interest in my progress in the following days, but there was nothing more I could add until I had the tests. One afternoon, Jacqui and I returned from a drive to find an old footy mate, Kevin Walters, had dropped by to ask if I wanted any company and, if I did, it might be a good idea to meet at Allan Langer's restaurant — Moo Bar at Caloundra — to 'see the boys'. Initially, I didn't feel like stepping out, but after a while I thought, 'Why not? I already have a dinner planned with family and friends at another restaurant around 8.30pm, so why not go for just a little while?'

I arrived about 4pm and it was a beautiful summer's day. Typically, Alf — with a sly grin — offered me a beer as soon as I got there. 'Thanks but no thanks,' I told him. It had been years since I'd got on the drink with the boys; he knew that but he was probably trying to get even with me for the nights that Gene Miles and I had done a job on him as our 'welcome' to the Queensland State of Origin team. Unfortunately, the little bastard succeeded. After watching him and Kevvie enjoy their drinks, I thought, 'Why not join them for a couple? If I'm going to have brain surgery and be cooped up in a hospital ward for days or maybe weeks, I might as well give myself the liberty of having a beer beforehand.' It didn't eventuate as a good idea.

Some time later, I discovered Alf was drinking half Scotch and water while Kevvie was drinking light beer as I'd tucked into Coronas. Jacqueline came to get me several hours later, after I hadn't called to be picked up or walked the 400 metres back home. For someone who was only going to be an hour or so, I was pretty late. To say I wasn't in the best shape would be an understatement: I was legless; the first time I'd been drunk for a long, long while — I'm guessing 10 years.

I went to dinner and hadn't been in the restaurant long when I noticed former Parramatta and Wigan rugby league coach John Monie at the next table. On my way to the toilet I stopped to say hello, but did so with a few expletives, which is far from usual for me in public and it certainly didn't suit the occasion. With a couple of minutes to steady myself, I realised I owed John's table an apology. I explained that I'd just had my first drink for ages and how Alf and Kevvie had set me up. Knowing the two of them quite well, John just laughed and accepted the apology, which I appreciated.

That was the last drink I had … both that night and until this day.

I woke up next morning with the biggest headache I'd had in years. Little did I know it would pale into insignificance compared to one that would come along about two months later.

I'd been on annual leave from work through to the New Year since my on-air seizure, but that had elapsed and, after talking to Andrew Slack, it was agreed I'd go back to work for a week before heading down to Melbourne. Rather than it being a painful trip down memory lane, I felt quite comfortable going back to Nine and working away from the camera, although my confidence had been severely dented. I received another couple of requests for an interview, but I declined, again stating that it was of no use before my visit to Melbourne.

In the next few weeks I suffered a couple of 'turns', again a few days apart, but the increased periods of rest I'd been enjoying seemed to have ensured they were becoming less frequent than previously. The day to go to Melbourne finally came and I was naturally quite nervous. We settled into our hotel a few kilometres from the Austin and found the nearest train station. It was good to find that travelling to and from the hospital would be easy for Jacqui, with a station virtually right outside the front door.

My first appointment was on Friday 9 February, when I was told I'd been scheduled for a cat scan, which I'd had dozens of times before, thanks to too many head knocks playing footy. Later that day, Lane Calcutt rang to tell of the passing of legendary rugby league referee Barry Gomersall, and asked me to make a comment to camera. It put a sad end to what had been an enjoyable day, which included a nice lunch and shopping in Melbourne, always a favourite pastime of Jacqui's.

Before I had to return to the hospital to become a resident for a while, we took the opportunity to take a two-day trip along the Great Ocean Road. For years I'd dreamed about travelling down the famous coastal stretch and admiring the 12 Apostles, and when it came true I wasn't disappointed. Despite inclement weather, we found ourselves amongst hundreds of tourists, and as is the case with the world's most famous landmarks, I never got tired of the view; it was spectacular. But visiting famous scenery didn't end there. After returning to Melbourne and freshening up, we headed to Lygon Street for dinner to a restaurant Lane had recommended, and it soon became clear why it had his stamp of approval. The size of the meal ensured that walking home after dinner was a necessity. The only moment of discomfort during a wonderful evening came from Calcutt minutes before our arrival at our hotel, when he suggested the hospital food may not quite be up to the standard we'd just enjoyed. Each time Jacqui and I returned to Melbourne from then on, we went back to the restaurant and repeated the walk to the hotel. However, the delicious meal that first night was the last big feed I was to have for a while.

Usually I'm a light eater at breakfast, enjoying cereal and a cup of coffee at the most, and 12 February 2007 wasn't any different. Perhaps it was because of the huge dinner the night before, or maybe because I was a little nervous about what lay ahead, but I had little appetite. I thought I was in a fairly comfortable mood, but following our arrival at the hospital, I started to get a little edgy. I'd noticed two men getting into the lift in the car park at the same time as us, and while it was quite natural for them to also get off up at the ground floor, they followed Jacqui and me across the hospital entrance to another set of lifts. We had to navigate a large crowd of people and, after realising we'd gone the wrong way, we back-tracked to the lift we'd just stepped out of. As I pressed the 'up' button, the same two men rushed into the lift just before the doors closed.

I became curious about why they seemed to be following us and my growing suspicion increased further when neither of them even looked to see if the button for their floor had been pushed. When the lift stopped at the floor I originally pushed I didn't move, waiting to see if they did. Just as the doors began to close, I pushed the button to reopen the doors. The pair followed us out and then tagged us down several corridors before entering a room where all epilepsy patients had to complete the paperwork for their upcoming tests. There I noticed one had a large bag that I believed to be carrying camera equipment, while the other bloke appeared to have a pad in his hands.

That was enough for me. I thought they had to be from the media, but just when I was about to protest their presence I was called over by the staff to book in for my tests. After filling in all the paperwork for my admission, I turned to notify Jacqueline that we were ready to go and the first face I saw was that of the man who'd been following us. He had joined me at the counter, but to my surprise, he began advising staff that he was there to help check his son in for the same tests I was about to have myself. I felt like a real goose, and after we transferred to the ward together, we introduced ourselves. It was Ron Shaw and his son Steve from Darwin.

I was admitted to an individual room, which just happened to be alongside Steve's, and shown the hi-tech monitoring equipment that was going to track my 'behaviour' 24/7, including an overhead camera centred upon the room. I saw a chair and plenty of electrical medical monitoring equipment … but there was no bed. I thought perhaps it was being replaced after a previous patient had left, but I was told that the chair was my 'home' for the next 10 days or so. 'All day?' I objected. 'Shit; that's a long time to sit on your arse!'

I thought that at least they'd bring in a bed for me to get a solid night's sleep. Wrong. In fact, I'd be spending all that time being monitored 24 hours a day in what resembled a single lounge chair. I was informed that the next week to 10 days was all about being uncomfortable and being denied sleep for long periods. To help that occur, that meant no mattress in the room. But there was a reason for that; in denying sleep, the brain would become very tired and stressed, and this was instrumental in bringing on seizures. That made sense. I knew that a long night out, or being forced to get up early for a couple of days in a row, would almost certainly bring on seizures.

I had a mass of attachments glued to my skull, each wire there to map any electrical currents generated in my brain which may cause seizures. I was advised that an alarm was clearly available to notify staff, should a seizure be about to take place.

It wasn't just the sleep patterns I was to be denied; I was informed that a bed pan was on hand to help me go to the loo and I'd be bathed every day in the chair. 'No way,' I decided. Instead, each day I'd get up out of the chair, guide the mass of wiring attached to my head across the room and open the bathroom door. The funny thing was that, after stepping inside, I couldn't quite make it all the way into the shower. So I'd lift the nozzle from the wall and hydrate my necessary parts. It meant plenty of water went all over the floor, but after I got out, my feet were able to push the towels around to mop up the water. I knew this would be a long and frustrating period, but it was better than not washing properly at all or getting a bed bath! It remained Jacqui's daily point of laughter.

Another thing I was to go without was a blanket to cover myself with when I did doze off. I was told that was to avoid concealing any body movements while I was being observed, especially if I was to have a seizure.

On day three of the scans, there was a mood-changing experience. It was mid-afternoon and I was watching television while Jacqueline was reading a book. I began to feel a little uneasy and knew something was about to occur. The tingles started to go through my body; I knew I was having a turn and looked around to push the alarm.

I recall grabbing the buzzer and also trying to inform Jacqueline. I thought she jumped up after noticing me trying to alert her, and yelled out to the nurses, two of whom came into the room to assist me. I guessed I was in a state of confusion for about a minute and a half to two minutes. But my recollections weren't quite what occurred. Jacqueline later told me I got it right about the two nurses, but another five or six entered the room before a whole host of doctors appeared to get a close-up of what was happening with my seizure. They stayed until it was agreed that everything was starting to settle. I can't remember any of that, I was 'off the air', but my wife informed me that it lasted around four to five minutes.

It was a seizure that fitted into the fairly strong category, and after being cleared by the doctors, I was placed on a portable hospital bed and wheeled away for a PET scan, which takes place immediately after a seizure to map brain patterns. 'You beauty,' I thought. 'Back on a comfortable bed at last!' It was probably the only time I actually felt glad to have a seizure! From there I was taken down a couple of floors to be mapped again, with the scans lasting about an hour and a half. As usual, I felt a little drained after the incident and had a nap during the later moments inside the radiology department. But there were plenty of things that went through my mind as the scanner moved overhead. The length of my seizure was obviously far longer than I'd suspected and it made me wonder whether many I'd had over the years were too.

It was an experience I underwent twice more during my stay, although I wasn't required to be scanned after those seizures, because the results of the first one had provided doctors with an almost perfect map of the positioning and size of the pertinent part of the brain that needed attention.

If having to go through enforced seizures and sitting in that bloody chair day and night was tough for me, life wasn't much fun for Jacqueline either. She was based in a fold-out bed at the side of the room, and every day she'd rise, have a shower, and return some of the calls and texts she'd received, to update our friends on how things were going. Often she'd then walk down to the nearby shops or catch a train to Ivanhoe just a couple of stops away to grab some delicious sandwiches, chocolates and biscuits for us. A board game or two were added as my hospital stint progressed and, while they certainly broke the boredom, I don't recall becoming an Einstein in the games department.

You find an interesting range of people among hospital staff and normally there is always one colourful character. In the case of the Austin it was a wardsman called Les, who made a point of dropping into my room every time he was nearby, to bag the hell out of me or drop a funny line. One of his main targets was the daily television news; his versions of events were far more interesting, if far fetched, than the actual story. Les had me in stitches some days and I'd like to think I gave him as good as I copped when I was feeling sharp enough. I expected him to ease off a little as the operation day neared, but he only appeared to increase his output. When I went back for my 12-month check-up, I ran into Les and asked him why he went out of his way to indulge in the rather cutting, but humorous, banter, and he told me it was to reduce the pressure on patients who might have been nervous about their daunting upcoming treatments. I then noticed him move through a dozen other rooms where his dose of humour was well appreciated. Every time I go back for a check-up I try to catch up with him … and his insults.

Next day, I was briefed by Professor Berkovic about the extensive scanning that would determine if I was suitable for the operation that I desperately hoped could change my life. My main point of concern was whether my short-term memory would improve. It had been driving me mad for some time, but I was told that while it most likely wouldn't get any better, it shouldn't get any worse.

Naturally, I'll never forget the date — 18 February 2007: D-Day. The results of my tests had been put in front of a group of over 130 medical staff, who'd analysed and discussed them before conferring on a decision about whether I was suitable for the operation. It was a meeting that lasted four hours. Shortly afterwards, Professor Berkovic came around to my room and indicated that he wanted to meet with Jacqui and me to discuss my future. Mitchell was in the room with his girlfriend and one of his friends, Josh, after just arriving from Brisbane. Unfortunately, as I've mentioned, Lincoln couldn't be there as he was under his own bit of pressure while auditioning for a role in *Home and Away*.

Sam asked if Jacqui and I wanted the kids to leave the room while he presented his findings, but I had no reason to clear the room; I had nothing to hide from them. Sam went on to inform me that the results of the tests were clear. There was some discussion over apparent scarring in one area of the brain, but it was impossible to conclude that it was caused by blunt force trauma through playing football; in any case, they felt surgery would provide a successful outcome. He told me that it was now time for me to decide my path: surgery, or to attempt to control my seizures through different forms of medication.

Most people went home to discuss the issue with their family with plenty of time for consideration. We'd already received, in writing, details of likely results of the surgery which was that 60 per cent have no subsequent seizures, 20 per cent had far fewer seizures, and 20 per cent are no better off. The risks involved were listed as '1 per cent serious complications such as stroke (during surgery), infection or death; 3 per cent chance of disruption to sight, enough to preclude a return to driving', plus there is some risk of paralysis to one side of the body, loss of speech and serious memory loss. It also stated that there was no expectation that current memory function would improve. So heavy was the demand for surgery it sometimes took up to six months before an operation was available anyway.

I saw no need to hesitate; I interrupted his explanation about the need for deep and extended thought and discussion and said, 'Look, I'm going ahead with the surgery, Sam. I've already been down every other path. To be honest, I'm not interested in any other option.'

Despite Jacqueline having been beside me throughout my eight days in the Austin and having had ample opportunities to talk it over with her, I'd spent hours considering the options to myself, especially when she was asleep or had gone to have lunch with the boys, and had made my decision. Once again, Sam brought up the value of having time to consider the options; again I insisted that the medical team had my full support. 'I'm going ahead with it and that's all there is to it.' He then advised us that a position on the surgery list had become available two days later. *Two days!!* That surprised me greatly. A position had 'become available'? Did someone change their mind or had the position eventuated in more tragic circumstances? We never found the answer, nor did we pursue it.

It might have been rude not to ask Jacqueline's opinion as she sat next to me, but I knew she was all for it; she didn't want to go through months of consideration either. We'd done that years earlier when considering the future for Jamie-Lee; spending over two years to-ing and fro-ing over whether to allow her to have the cochlear implant. My decision was much simpler than that.

I felt relieved rather than anxious, but the good mood didn't last long. Steve, the bloke who I'd suspiciously thought was a journalist the first day I walked into the hospital, had just received the results about his suitability for the brain surgery. He'd received a 'negative'. His dad was shattered — he came into my room to say goodbye and broke into tears. He was angry and disappointed. Not at the doctors, just the results; he couldn't understand why his son hadn't been given a fair go in life. I couldn't give him an explanation.

Steve, who I'd got to know reasonably well during our stay, was a lovely bloke, a real gentleman. He appeared to be handling the news better than his father, saying he'd been down this road — of seeking a better treatment — plenty of times before; it was just time to go back home to Darwin and get on with life. Steve had suffered epilepsy since birth, but after finding the love of his life, he was married and suddenly his life changed. He never had a single seizure from that day ... until his wife contracted a fatal disease and passed away six months after their wedding. Upon her death, Steve returned to his routine of daily seizures. His and his dad's departure was a very sad event. I kept in contact with Steve for a while and his battle with regular seizures continues. I think of him often and how he is getting on.

While Steve's news flattened me, it made me more conscious that I was a lucky one. And, with little notice, I was getting ready to go under the knife within 48 hours. Unlike others in the Austin hospital who'd had far more serious scenarios to contend with, I didn't have a life-threatening condition, and I was conscious of that; but it was still a life-altering procedure and I was anxious and uncertain of what my existence would be like when I woke from the anaesthetic.

The time had come — what I'd dismissed as the absolute last resort was now about to become a reality.

ANOTHER PERSPECTIVE

Professor Peter Silburn, Consultant Neurologist

When I first saw Wally in professional consultation, he was having multiple non-convulsive seizures whilst he was talking throughout the appointment. He was having blank spells, picking up late on the flow of the conversation, was seemingly withdrawn and somewhat anxious. Jacqui was appropriately attentive by his side in concerned support.

At the time Wally was taking significant doses of antiepileptic drugs which were not holding his fits at bay. A neurological colleague found a site in the brain causing the epilepsy, and sometime ago rightly suggested that Wally needed an operation to remove the causative area.

Wally knew he was in trouble and the question remained as to why he had baulked at the neurologist's advice. Persistence and determination are the stuff of great champions and perhaps these outstanding qualities of Wally Lewis, which he helped instil into a generation of Queensland footballers, was holding him back? Not so; it was the core human quality of worrying about the consequences of such an operation, particularly its potential risks and losses if such an operation went wrong.

Wally had seen another sporting champion, an Australian football captain from another code, who had trouble with speech after a similar operation. Wally wanted to and needed to continue working as a sports journalist and presenter and was worried any effect on his speech would end his career and his ability to support his family.

With Jacqui's and his family's help we worked through his mental and emotional block. They decided to go ahead with surgery and went to the outstanding Australian Epilepsy Centre in Melbourne and as such avoided the feverish rugby league media of Queensland and New South Wales. We reasoned it would give him a better chance of a less pressured recovery. Really he just needed a different helping hand.

The rest is history. Wally's story is a testament to the perseverance of the Lewis family. It is a successful story of a great champion and a champion family and is best told by them.

TWELVE

BRAIN SURGERY

IT may sound a little corny, but after waking on the day I was scheduled for surgery, I felt like a gun-slinger from an old western movie who'd just watched the sun rise on the day he was to have a shoot-out in the main street at high noon.

Before we departed our hotel room, Jacqueline started to talk her head off and I was left wondering just who between us was more nervous. We arrived at the hospital around 10am to undergo the usual pre-op basics, and from there it was a matter of listening to the clock tick.

We waited for about 45 minutes and Mitchell and Lincoln were very talkative. Then the nurse arrived to tell me to don the gown for surgery and get ready to be taken around to theatre; it was time for the operation. The atmosphere changed instantly. Jacqueline gave the tissues a workout, the boys went quiet and I wasn't much better. The trepidation was contagious; the mood sombre.

Linc started to calm his mother and, just before I was wheeled away on the trolley, I grabbed Mitch, pulled him to the side, gave him a hug and said, 'It's not likely, but if something does go wrong or I don't turn out to be the full quid, you have to take control and look after your mother and sister,' before kissing his forehead. I don't really recall what, if anything, he said in reply but we looked into each other's eyes, feeling, 'Surely it will never come to that, but … you never know for sure.'

Jacqueline was still shedding tears as I was wheeled into surgery, where my first challenge occurred. In the operating theatre, I met again with the surgeon, Professor Gavin Fabinyi, and his assistant, as well as the anaesthetist. Professor Fabinyi's assistant was a Queenslander and we'd previously shared plenty of jokes during the pre-surgery tests and the results. While the anesthetist prepared to inject me, I told her that going under the knife was a fairly common thing for me, and I used to joke with the fellow in Brisbane who regularly worked on my injections about how long I'd last before lapsing into unconsciousness. You'd be asked to count down from ten seconds to zero with the belief no one would go close to finishing the count. The highest mark I'd reached was counting down to seven seconds, although I believe on a couple of occasions he'd started to insert the drug a little earlier than he indicated just to win the 'contest' (that I could outlast the 10-second count). However, this time I didn't get to even start the countdown; I don't know whether she injected the drip before I looked or whether I was a little too nervous.

The operation — called a temporal lobe resection — lasted just under four hours. It began with having a line drawn on my head to mark out the incision. Following that the bone was cut to gain access to the brain and part of the temporal lobe tissue — where the memory is stored — was removed.

Although I was very heavily sedated, apparently I saw Jacqui and Mitch after they were invited into the post-op ward following the operation; I don't remember it at all. Jacqueline claimed I kissed her and said, 'I love you,' which would have been the perfect first words for a husband to say, but I'll never know whether it was true or just her interpretation of my mumbling!

My first recollection wasn't until very late that night. Soon after I was wheeled away into the recovery room, Gavin, Jacqueline, Mitchell and Lincoln spoke to journalists at a media conference and it must have been quite settling for Jacqui and the boys to hear the surgeon declare, 'Everything went well.'

When I woke a couple of hours later, I felt like I'd been hit with an axe. It was the most intense headache I'd ever experienced and I asked the nurse to administer further painkilling 'syrup'. I woke again a couple of hours after that, and after another dose of pain relief I eventually got quite a good night's sleep. When I woke the next morning, I was apparently quite confused and a bit distressed that Jacqueline wasn't in the room and I asked the nurses over and over again where she was. I didn't remember that she wouldn't be staying overnight with me as the post-op rooms were off-limits, and that she'd be visiting during the allocated hours. Recalling the most basic detail was a major problem for quite a few weeks.

When I saw Jacqui that morning she'd become fairly quiet, again something not natural for her, and she dropped the volume of her speaking so as not to aggravate my constant throbbing head. My parents, June and Jim, arrived the next day with my sister Jeannie, and it was obvious Jacqui hadn't given them 'softly, softly' tips; still, it was great to see them and you could tell they were greatly relieved that I seemed okay. As usual, the old man didn't get too many words in, with Mum, my sister and wife in the same room, and he was left shaking his head on plenty of occasions at how much they could talk. There was a bit of conversation between me and Dad, but I was conscious of how slowly I was speaking, which worried me. Hearing my slow speech must have been hard for him.

The headaches, more powerful than I'd ever had before the surgery, continued for probably three days; they were 'bell ringers'. If there was the slightest indication that another one was coming on I'd press the buzzer for a nurse to get another injection to dim the pain.

Gradually, over the next 72 hours, the pain level went down and I was weaned onto lower dosages of painkillers. I was also told I no longer had to take four different drugs twice daily; my intake of Keppra and Topomax was to end. Also departing from my daily existence, thankfully, was the drip that was inserted into my penis to urinate through. It felt like they were dragging a barbed wire fence out of me! I rate that the most uncomfortable moment of my life; save for the headaches I experienced after the surgery!

I was released from the Austin after five days but I had to stay in Melbourne and not venture too far from the hospital, in case any post-operative distress occurred. I also had to return to the hospital five days later for final assessment. I'd been well looked after there and the pampering only continued 'outside' following my discharge.

My head was heavily bandaged for 10 days after the operation and it wasn't until I removed it that I saw a massive scar, about 32 centimetres long, that travelled from the middle of my forehead, above the left eye, back through the hairline in a semi-circular fashion before sliding down the front side of my ear and stopping level with the canal — almost the shape of a question mark. I wasn't a pretty sight. But, inside, I felt good knowing that every single indication was that the surgery had gone as well as could be expected — and if Gavin Fabinyi and Sam Berkovic believed that, that was as good a recommendation as I wanted.

I felt tired and sore and a bit unsteady, but I mostly felt relieved and quite excited. I was confident I'd begun a new, better life. After sinking so low a couple of months earlier, going through the uncomfortable days of trying to instigate seizures, and the anxiousness of being booked into the surgery on such short notice, I could hope that seizures would be in the past tense in my life.

Dick 'Tosser' Turner had called on one of our former Maroons stars, John Ribot, to ensure my discharge would be more than comfortable. That was typical of good old Richard, whose friendship was priceless to me. Over the years, I'd seen Tosser ensure his troops were well looked after and he could inevitably negotiate a 'deal' for our benefit. On one occasion, council workers in Sydney had suddenly appeared on the scene in a park about 25 metres from the back of our hotel just hours before kick-off in a series-deciding State of Origin match at the SCG and were making a hell of a racket. Tosser went out and appealed to the workers to down tools for a while so we could get some much needed pre-match rest. They weren't interested until Tosser placed his hand into his pocket, pulled out a wad of notes and asked the council boys if they'd like to extend their lunch break and dine out in style. They weren't seen again. We won the match that night.

On several occasions, Tosser was also responsible for flying the wife and kids or parents of a new inclusion into the Queensland team to Sydney or Brisbane for the game if they were struggling financially. He was one of nature's gentlemen; probably the finest I ever came across. It was a sad day when he passed away in June 2008, aged 76.

On Tosser's suggestion, 'Reebs', who boasted plenty of experience with Melbourne's lifestyle, having spent several years as CEO of the Melbourne Storm, had arranged that Jacqui and I spend the next five days at 'acceptable' accommodation — the Grand Hyatt, arguably Melbourne's finest hotel, where the manager really looked after us. We were joined by Tosser and his wife Jan, Gene Miles and his wife Debbie, 'Reebs' and former FOGS boss Alan Graham. It was a wonderful gesture and great to see them all — even though I wasn't looking or feeling my best.

We were staying on the 23rd floor with a panoramic city view, but spent plenty of time gazing out over even better scenery in the penthouse restaurant. While it probably bored the shit out of the others to just sit around, I was comfortable just sitting there not doing much. Tea became my regular 'brew' from that time. Since the operation I hadn't had one cup of coffee, and that was strange; normally I'd consume six or seven every day. When Jacqui ordered me a coffee the day after the operation, the smell of it just didn't appeal to me. I asked for tea and Jacqui laughed. I became a devotee of English Breakfast tea; Jacqui served me herbal tea once but it tasted dreadful.

Tosser, Reebs, Gene and the girls went home after ensuring I was more than relaxed for the next few days, but the company didn't dry up. My former business partner and team-mate Peter O'Callaghan arrived with two of his daughters, Annie and Lizzie, who is my god-daughter.

'Cal' is a trusted mate and has been for a long time. I first met him the day after my Valleys team had won the under-18 grand final in 1977. Our team was celebrating in the club the next day, and upon arriving at the bar, I saw this bloke who was in worse condition than me and my team-mates — and that was saying something. After ordering a round of drinks, I found myself trapped in a headlock which was only released when the bloke told me he was too thirsty to continue. He introduced himself and from that moment Cal and I became very close. In fact, the child whose birth he was celebrating that day, Ben O'Callaghan, was page boy at my wedding seven years later.

We'd often enjoyed many a drink together, had been partners in a hotel in Toowoomba and just good, trusted mates. His presence in Melbourne was very welcome, although not for too long. Cal had organised to take Jacqui, me and his daughters out for dinner. I still wasn't particularly hungry, but getting out of the room was great. He led the way to his selected restaurant, and after five minutes or so of walking I was asking how much further we had to go. A further 10 minutes into the trip I was still wondering, and asking; after another five minutes of navigating pavement after pavement and intersection after intersection I felt like I'd run a marathon and didn't mind telling Cal. Eventually we arrived at the casino, where we enjoyed a wonderful meal.

When it came time to walk back home, Cal started to laugh. He wasn't going to put himself through the interrogation or the fatigue again and decided he'd have a punt and a night out with his daughters before getting a cab home, leaving Jacqui and me to hit the streets again alone. Despite not winning a cent at the casino, Cal says he laughed continuously all night, thinking of me struggling back to the hotel. I would have bitten his head off if he was there!

I was okay getting around Melbourne when Jacqui was there to navigate, but without her the next day, thanks to the state of my confused memory due to part of my brain having just been removed, it became quite an ordeal. We'd gone to a huge shopping mall to buy gifts for the kids, and while she was there, Jacqui dropped into a hairdressing salon to make an appointment. She'd been tending to me so constantly for the previous couple of months she really hadn't had a chance to get her hair done, and men know how that can tend to upset women! The hairdresser had a vacancy right then, but Jacqui was hesitant to leave me alone. I told her to grab the chance and I'd walk back up the hill to the hotel.

I walked out and set off on the path I recognised as the way 'home' — probably not much more than half a kilometre, I thought. The street I'd targeted to make a turn was, I'd guessed, about two hundred metres up the street. After 30 minutes of searching, I still hadn't found it and started to panic. Several times, I thought I recognised the right way, only to head down another wrong path. I couldn't even remember the name of the hotel, and despite pulling the keys out of my pocket with the address marked on it, it didn't last long in my memory. Even asking someone the way proved too difficult; I went to ask several people but each time withdrew my request halfway through my question and set off to find the hotel myself. Eventually I took the correct path to finally get to my destination after a fair bit of stress. While I wasn't quite in a state of panic, I was very anxious and frustrated. The walk had obviously knocked me around a bit, and after lying on the bed, I must have dozed off. But not for long ...

Jacqueline returned and looked to be in the same state of panic that I had been in an hour or so earlier. She was furious with the hairdresser's work and the price didn't amuse her either; it cost well over $300 and three hours in the chair. Added to that, she hated the hairstyle. It was probably the only thing we didn't enjoy about this trip to Melbourne.

The following day we went back to the Austin, had one last check-in with Professor Berkovic and got the all-clear to return home, with an appointment booked for a check-up three months later.

Before we left, Jacqui organised a trip out to Melbourne Storm training just near Olympic Park, and we were received wonderfully by the Storm officials, before I went out onto the field to watch the team train. A few of the players came over to say hello, which was nice; and what made it even better was that they were all Queenslanders — Cameron Smith, Dallas Johnson, Billy Slater, Mick Crocker, Cooper Cronk and Greg Inglis.

A club official suggested we all have a photograph taken together; the toughest thing was trying to fit into the only Storm jersey available. It was a medium, apparently the same size worn by many of their stars on game day. It was extremely tight, which made it difficult for defending opponents to grab in a tackle.

After the shot was taken, the media manager instructed the photographer that the photo was for private use only, and I'd agreed to pose with the players under that condition. However, the next day it appeared in the *Herald Sun* in Melbourne, *The Daily Telegraph* in Sydney and the Brisbane *Courier-Mail*, with a small story and (in Melbourne) a photo of me putting on the jersey. I thought it was a low act and from then I decided I'd have no contact with any media other than my employer Channel 9. I was very upset.

My mood quickly changed when Jamie-Lee flew to Melbourne to join us for two or three days after being involved in a water polo training camp in Sydney. Jacqui had kept in constant contact with her so she was fully aware of my situation. During the camp she'd been vying for selection in the Australian water polo team while the rest of her family was in Melbourne, and that was obviously tough for her. While she is very determined in her sports, it was apparent that family distress had taken priority in her mind. She was cut from the squad and Jacqueline arranged for her to come to Melbourne to catch up with us, and for us to give her some much-needed love and support.

As we waited at the airport we thought she must have missed the flight; she was nowhere in sight as a parade of people came out of the arrival lounge from what was obviously a packed flight. Jacqui started to panic a little when ... she was second last off the flight, a long way behind the others. As soon as she saw us Jamie-Lee began crying, which is a very uncommon occurrence. Maybe it was because I had my head heavily bandaged, added to the fact that she had plenty of things on her mind. After listening to her on the trip back to our hotel, it was obvious she hadn't had a pleasant time in Sydney, and missing selection in the Australian side obviously disappointed her. But it was great to have her with us; even though — after we got back to our motel room and I took off the bandages for a short while — she thought her old man looked a bit scary with a big slit across the left side of his head.

We went in to the Austin for the farewell instructions from the medical staff and, finally, we were going back to Queensland. There was to be no physical activity and plenty of rest until at least my three-month check-up. When we arrived at Brisbane airport, we decided to slip out the back door just in case there may have been any media waiting. I didn't see any there as we departed in a cab, but upon arriving home Lane Calcutt was waiting with Drew Towson, Channel 9 Brisbane's head cameraman. This time I didn't want to front another news camera and I don't think I could have offered anything constructive anyway, so Jacqui did an interview. Lane requested a follow-up story but Jacqui insisted this was not to be 'a drama series' and we'd contact him after returning to Melbourne three months later. While I was obviously conscious that I was employed by Channel 9, and the station had been wonderful for me, I now needed lots of rest … privately.

What eventuated was very different to a peaceful time putting my feet up. Just when I thought the success of the operation would open up a far more pleasurable life, I was instead confronted by a whole new ordeal that sent me into a new depth of depression; enough for me to contemplate taking my life.

ANOTHER PERSPECTIVE

By Ben Dobson, reporter, Channel 9 Brisbane

When I began at Channel 9 in 1999, I would make it a priority to reminisce with Wally about the good old days of footy in the '80s. I loved hearing his stories about the games, the players and culture of the Brisbane rugby league scene but pretty soon Wally's remembrances seemed to have one thing in common: they were the same story. For reasons unbeknown at the time Wally kept reading the story from the same page, so to speak, and I'd sit there thinking to myself, 'Haven't I heard this just last week?'

I dismissed his memory loss as perhaps a knock too many to the head but as I got to know him and work closer with him, I noticed how easily he forgot menial tasks every day and how he had to use post-it notes to remind him to do things, like take his wallet home, buy lunch and ring so-and-so. More concerning was when you looked into his eyes; you'd capture a vacant stare, catatonic more than day-dreaming.

It's now a thing of the past.

He's a new person. His stories and memories are fresh and clear; he seldom repeats himself and he's alert and observant to everything around him.

Wow. What a transformation.

THIRTEEN

ROCK BOTTOM

FOR weeks I'd wondered why I so often felt upset; so utterly depressed and frustrated. My life had become Groundhog Day, the same routine every time I got out of bed, bound by the walls of our home. I needed constant baby-sitting, my short-term memory loss was driving me crazy, for no apparent reason I would cry and I'd also follow Jacqueline around like a mongrel dog and not know why. After a couple of months of this, I'd just had enough.

On several occasions when Jacqueline went to the shops and left me alone for short periods, I would walk down to the jetty out the back of our house. At first I'm sure it was just to enjoy the sea breeze and surroundings, but after a dozen or so visits I began to contemplate my future. Twice, that I can remember, I just decided I didn't want any more of my confined, confused daily life and ended up bawling my eyes out with my hands over my face, in the absolute depths of despair over what had happened to me. I thought of securing a heavy bag of rocks around my neck and diving from our pontoon into the canal.

I still don't know why I felt that way. It is obvious now I was suffering an uncontrollable bout of depression that was so black it just overtook me. Why didn't I go ahead with suicide? Again, I don't know why. It was like this spell had come over me and I couldn't work anything out about myself, but I do know I didn't want to continue any longer in that condition. Maybe it was the coward in me that stopped me taking the next step towards ending the misery; maybe it was a feeling deep below my depression that the pain I was going through was nothing compared to the pain I'd put others through if I was selfish and irrational enough to take my life. But what I do know is that I had never felt more miserable or so discontented with my life. And I just didn't know when or how I was going to crawl out of the dark cloud that seemed to have parked itself right over my head.

Eventually, while sitting there looking at the water, something inside me said, 'Don't you dare put your family through that pain after what they've already gone through.' Both my family and Jacqueline's had been hit by tragedy: 20 years earlier, my brother Eddie had been given 24 hours to live for several consecutive weeks after a serious car accident that killed two of his mates, but luckily he'd pulled through; while Jacqui's family had been struck with far sadder circumstances, with the loss of her brother John, who'd taken his life in 2000 at the age of 24.

I'd gradually been building to that terrible state of mind since the first few days after returning home from my hospital stint. As much as Jacqui and I took a real liking to Melbourne — it's a great cosmopolitan city with so many lifestyle attractions — it felt good to be back in Brisbane in familiar surroundings. But from that first day at our place, everything became so repetitive: I'd wake up, go downstairs, have a very light breakfast, see the kids off, then go into the lounge room and watch television. Strangely, I felt comfortable with that, especially watching TV for hours, which got me out of Jacqueline's way as well. Sometimes I'd have a 'kip' in the chair, but most of the time I enjoyed the shows I'd probably watched 40 years earlier with Dad at Cannon Hill, like *Gunsmoke*, *Bonanza*, *Maverick* and *The Untouchables*, as well as whatever was on the sports channels.

While very little changed each day I never felt bored, as I had very little urge to do much physically. Dr Marie O'Shea, who has the rather extensive title of deputy director of clinical neuro-psychology and clinical co-ordinator of the seizure, surgery and rehabilitation program at the Austin, had given us a fairly detailed plan of how my day should unfold, with basic rest and plenty of time set aside for sleep; and I had no problems adhering to that. I also had to have someone in my company 24/7.

Over the first few weeks I had plenty of family and friends come around to help Jacqueline, or provide her with a little bit of spare time if she needed to go to the shops or grab Jamie-Lee from school. Among those were my best man Brian Ball and groomsman Allan Mohle, who helped me get through plenty of my early days of recovery, despite probably being bored as buggery; but that's the kind of blokes they are.

Among the surprise visitors were former Queensland State of Origin forward Steve Jackson, another former Gold Coast Seagulls team-mate Paul Galea, Broncos and Queensland Origin legend Trevor 'The Axe' Gillmeister and Queensland's iconic fishing expert and *Coastwatch* guru Ken Brown, who I knew from my Channel 7 days. Their company must have been a relief for Jacqueline who was struggling to cope with my confused mind and neurotic behaviour. Former Valleys team-mate Tom Duggan also came around regularly and he did a bit of a minder's job; Jacqui would go and get some bread and milk at the shops and Tom would keep an eye on me. Another regular visitor was my former Fox Sports partner and good mate John McCoy. Macca is the kind of bloke who is always in a good mood, always has a smile on his face, so his role was to entertain, which is a natural pastime for him. My long-time friend George Metzakis and former Queensland rugby union representative Nigel Holt were another two regular 'minders'.

It was wonderful to hear from so many old football mates and two regular callers on the phone were former Queensland halfbacks Greg Oliphant and Barry Muir, which I appreciated, plus guys I played with like Steve Mortimer, Brett Kenny and Greg Conescu, and many others, including Cathy Freeman, Channel 9's Eddie McGuire, Cameron Williams, John Raper, Jeff Thomson, Ken Arthurson, Ray Phillips, Graham Lowe, Robyn Tallis (Gorden's sister), Rick Grossman from the Hoodoo Gurus, New Zealand's league nut Peter 'The Mad Butcher' Leitch and my old mate Mark 'Mullet' Ella.

Jacqueline had been looking after me like a live-in nurse for months, but there were plenty of things she needed to catch up on, particularly spending some time with Jamie-Lee and helping her with getting to school or training or just going to a party on the weekend. So she began to go out a little more, and when she left the house and Mitchell or Lincoln weren't around, she would arrange for me to be looked after by my dad Jim, my brother Scott or Jacqui's father and brother, both called Bruce, or my brother-in-law Mark Wilson. But it must have been trying for them at times having an absolute scatterbrain on their hands.

I knew it would take some time for my memory to recover fully, but I was starting to have a massive inability to recall anything at all — and that really concerned me. A definite low came one day when I'd settled into the lounge chair for my morning ritual — watching reruns of *Gunsmoke* and *Maverick*, before switching over to the sports channels while enjoying a cup of tea. Yes — I was still drinking tea.

This day, *Gunsmoke* had just finished and I got up to get something out of the kitchen, but after leaving the chair and walking past the fridge I couldn't remember what I'd walked in there for. I went back into the lounge, and sat down once again, before remembering about 20 minutes later what it was I wanted. I walked into the kitchen, but again when I arrived I couldn't recall my reason for going there. After re-entering the lounge room I started to make a joke about it, but just a few minutes later I remembered the reason again. I got out of the chair and said to my father-in-law, Bruce, 'I'll probably forget this time too,' and duly did. Bruce said it wasn't anything to worry about as he suffered the same problem every day. 'It's just something that happens when you get older … aw, well, not that you're old or anything.' His bit of humour broke my anxiety at least, but it didn't last long. It wasn't just frustrating me; I had a great fear that was what my memory was going to be like for the rest of my life.

Finally, when I went back to the kitchen and took something out of the fridge, I noticed my hands were shaking a little. In the days that followed, they were rattling more than trembling. But that wasn't the only disturbing feature about what was happening to me; if a knife was dropped or a cup hit another when placed into the sink, I'd jump; even the slightest noise frightened me.

A few days later I was in the kitchen with my sons when Lincoln twice asked me what was wrong. 'I'm fine, mate,' I apparently answered (a lot of this is going by the memory of others because it's all a haze to me). After further questioning I again reassured him I was okay, and asked why he wanted to know; he looked at me really concerned. It was only when I walked into the bathroom a little while later and looked in the mirror that I discovered why the boys were so concerned. I was crying — bawling my eyes out — and had no idea that I was doing it, or why. My immediate thoughts were, 'What the hell are you crying for, you dickhead?' But I couldn't stop it.

I'd started to feel confident enough for Jacqueline to go down to the local shops and leave me briefly by myself. But she'd only be gone two or three minutes (it seemed a lot longer to me) and I'd be parked at the front door nervously waiting for her return. One time she travelled up to the local hot bread kitchen, and as usual she got into a conversation with the girls who worked there, which always proved a little hard to escape. When she got back about 25 minutes later I was sitting around in tears, which naturally shocked her. At first she thought I may have suffered my first seizure since the operation, but that wasn't the case. The biggest issue was that I had no idea why I was crying.

It was during that period that I bordered on becoming suicidal. I was at my worst probably two months after the operation. I'd spoken to Penny Kincade, the Neurology and Epilepsy Liaison Nurse at the Austin, about how I was feeling. Penny had been a tower of strength since our first day of contact four months earlier, educating us on the process of surgery and the recovery, and one thing she insisted was that whenever I had thoughts of suicide or just felt extremely low, to consult my doctors instantly. But I kept my suicide thoughts from Jacqui and the kids;

she'd been through enough with her brother and I didn't want to put her into a spin. However, when I spoke to her, Penny rang Jacqui, who immediately sought the assistance of staff at the Austin Hospital. They warned her that sometimes things can go a little amiss for a few months after the brain surgery and my depression was not unusual.

I snapped out of the self-pity long enough to realise I needed to consult the people who'd been of great assistance throughout the whole campaign. Firstly, I spoke to my local GP, Dr John Craven, who I'd been visiting for about 13 years and knew all about my battles, and who I consider a good friend. He contacted Professor Peter Silburn, the man who'd directed me to Melbourne for surgery, and after their discussion John prescribed Cipramil, an anti-depressant that also assists with anxiety. I was told the tablets can play a fairly strong role straight away, and was directed to begin taking half a tablet a day. They worked instantly and the dosage was raised to one a day and my mood lifted significantly.

But while my mental state finally seemed on the mend, physically another shock was just around the corner. Jamie-Lee had gained selection in a representative netball team and was involved in a two-day carnival at which the state champions would be crowned. It gave

Jacqueline an opportunity to provide proud support, but it would also be the first time that she'd spent a lengthy period away from me. So it was organised for me to spend the day at 'the outlaws', with her parents Bruce and Kathy. Upon my arrival at their place, Jacqueline's mother had a big Sunday breakfast waiting, partnered by a tall cup of tea. Another session viewing the favourite old television programs followed and I was feeling nice and content until …

Just as lunch was served, I started to feel a bit dicey in the stomach. Within half an hour I was buckling over in agony and minutes later I had no doubt what was occurring: I had kidney stones. I'd suffered from them before, and when we arrived at my GP's surgery, the doctor advised me that I could go to the hospital but as I'd discovered previously, it really wouldn't be of any benefit. I knew it would be a case of just going home and riding it out. Earlier, I'd asked Kathy not to call Jacqueline and that Bruce and I would contact her after we'd seen the doctor. I should have known better: Kathy had rung Jacqueline as we drove out the front gates to head to the doctor's. Jacqui arrived at her parents' house to check out my condition after our return. Bruce suggested that, if we were ever going to rob a bank, not to tell Kathy as she'd have the police waiting before we got there. Upon reflection, I suppose she didn't really know what was wrong and decided to warn Jacqui just in case.

A few days later my kidney stones had settled down but my eyes started playing up. It was 8.30am and I'd just got up after an uncomfortable night. I started reading the paper, which is virtually a daily habit for me in the first hour of being awake, but I began to struggle to make out the words clearly. That wasn't unusual; I'd normally wipe my eyes and focus on something else for a minute, then return to the paper and all would be fine. But this time my vision didn't appear to get any clearer. I thought perhaps this was an indication that reading specs were finally in order, but as I looked out across the canal I noticed the scenery had a yellow-orange colour and everything seemed a little bright. About 15 minutes later I was struggling to see anything clearly at all. Jacqueline and I were both worried as we'd heard about difficulties with vision in the post-operative recovery period, so she got straight onto the phone to notify Dr Craven. We were immediately given a referral to head into the city and visit a specialist, but despite a lengthy check later that day he diagnosed that my eyes were fine and it may just have been 'one of those things'. My vision slowly started to return to normal over the next few hours, which was a massive relief; the cause of my troubles was never detected.

Only a week or so later I had a second opportunity to step out of the house in over two months, when I took up an invitation to visit Ken Brown's house at bayside Wynnum in Brisbane. I felt I needed some quality time away from home where I could gain some confidence, and after arriving at his place Browny and I sat in the living room having a cuppa — tea, of course — while talking about footy.

Ken had a small dog in the room, and a few minutes later it appeared to me that he was having a bit of a scratch, which was nothing unusual. Then it got a bit more animated and was brushing against my leg and I wondered what the hell it was doing. I asked Browny what was wrong with his mutt and he replied with an hysterical laugh, 'Stuff you, King — you've come around here and given my dog epilepsy.' I thought he was having a joke … until I looked down to see the dog's front legs out to the side, flicking uncontrollably. I couldn't believe it. Next thing, his wife Shelly rushed the dog off to the vet. Ken had been deadly serious about his dog having epilepsy (although he was joking about how he contracted it). I had no idea dogs could suffer the condition!

While my life had become pretty much a daily ritual of repetition — breakfast, read the paper, watch the same shows on TV, sit out the back, more TV, a couple of naps and rarely leaving the house — there was one thing that did change over the first few weeks at home: my waistline. All my shorts became far too big for me, except for a few old ones I'd just about given up hope of ever fitting into again. A check on the scales indicated that my weight had dropped from 97 kilos down to 90. It continued to fall, and after another couple of months reached 84 kilos.

I just had no appetite and was eating little more each day than a piece of toast, maybe a sandwich and picking at my dinner. I was doing nothing physical other than walking a few paces around the house, so my body wasn't asking for any 'fuel' to burn off.

As late May 2007 approached, I was probably more nervous returning to the Austin Medical Centre for the three-month assessment than when I checked in for the operation. I feared that my explanation of the dramas at home and having had to add anti-depressant medication to my system may have been seen as a major hurdle.

At first we met with Penny Kincade and then Dr O'Shea and it was obvious that my mental status was the priority. Jacqueline and I described my troubles of the previous couple of months and, when it was time to talk to Professor Berkovic, I expected a bit of a grilling. But Sam's understanding of my recovery traumas boosted my confidence.

The second question of our meeting was to the point: 'Have you ever felt like taking your life?' I didn't hesitate for a minute to say yes, like I couldn't wait to get it out. He asked me whether those feelings happened at particular times of the day, but I told him there seemed to be no pattern. He assured me I wasn't the first, and wouldn't be the last, to go through such challenges.

A short-term plan was devised for altering the dosage of my medication and what exercise I could gradually embark on, as well as a target for my return to work. The good news was that I'd gone three months without suffering a seizure, gradually I was feeling stronger physically and, after those initial couple of months when I was at the end of my tether, I was feeling mentally stronger too.

The medical experts at the Austin seemed to think that if I took on these freshly laid-out measures, my recovery would progress fine. And they were to be proved right. Bit by bit, over quite a few months, I started to feel myself again and was able to leave those dark feelings of frustration and depression behind me.

ANOTHER PERSPECTIVE

By Lane Calcutt, Channel 9 Brisbane news reporter

As a work colleague of Wally's, and as a friend, I watched and agonised for him as he struggled through his on-air seizures, coped with the aftermath, and his obvious pain at the embarrassment he thought he'd brought to himself and Nine News. And as a journalist, Wally allowed me very privileged access, as he fought with the realisation that he had to do something incredibly traumatic to turn his life around.

Three moments during those weeks and months, before and after his operation, are indelibly etched. The first was several months before his surgery, when he was arguably at the most difficult time of his struggle.

Wally was at his Sunshine Coast holiday apartment. On my own, I dropped in. He was alone, and for a long time we sat on his back patio and discussed the decision he knew he had to make ... whether to go ahead and have that extraordinarily delicate surgery.

Wally was full of doubt. He knew the risks, knew the possible side effects if it went wrong. He showed me scientific articles, magazine stories of others who'd gone through the surgery; tales of triumph, some not so triumphant. I don't think he'd mind me saying — he was scared. But deep down, Wally knew he had to make the right decision for his family: wife Jacqui, his sons Mitch and Lincoln, and daughter Jamie-Lee.

It wasn't easy to watch him deal with it. We walked down to the beach and talked as friends. Something in me knew too that he'd give it a go. He wanted so much to give his family the peace of mind, and to be the husband and father he wanted them to have; that they deserved to have.

After travelling to Melbourne with Wally and Jacqui for the initial tests, I was there with cameraman John King when he underwent the operation. The next day brought the second 'moment' that lingers. Jacqui and the boys agreed to be interviewed about Wally's progress, just 24 hours after the operation.

When they walked into the room, after they'd seen Wally, the relief, the joy in their faces, was palpable. This massive weight had been lifted from their collective shoulders. It was hard to forget. They told me how Wally, in an 'un-Wally' moment, told them he loved them. Suddenly there was sunlight and hope in an otherwise gloomy Victorian capital.

Months later came the third special moment. Wally and Jacqui walked into the newsroom. That in itself was a giant step forward. He was there not to work, just to visit. He was relaxed, smiling, happy; clearly relieved. And he called me 'Nev' (Neville Nobody). Instantly, I knew Wally Lewis was back. He was a long way down that road to recovery.

Every day since has been a milestone.

I've been fortunate, and privileged, to be beside him during some of the bumpiest parts of that winding, at times painful, journey.

FOURTEEN

OUT OF THE FOG

I HAD never missed being at a State of Origin match —
as a player, coach, spectator or part of the working
media — since the first one back in July 1980. That was
78 straight Origin matches in Brisbane, Sydney,
Melbourne, even Long Beach, California.

I had felt like part of the furniture when it came to
Origin night at Suncorp Stadium and I loved every match
played there, irrespective of the result. I would suck up all
the atmosphere that is unique to Origin and it became a
part of me; it was such a familiar scene and I felt so
comfortable in that environment.

Having said that, it wasn't particularly enjoyable the first
time I went to watch an Origin match as an ex-
Queensland player, in 1992 — especially as New South
Wales won. Queensland lost that series 2–1 and that was
my toughest time as a FOG. I wished I was out there again

— I was still playing at the Gold Coast, and it was nagging away inside that maybe I could have helped us avoid defeat. I coached Queensland for the next two years, and, although we lost both series, that was a good way to replace the adrenalin rush I was missing. By the time 1995 came around and I had no direct involvement, I was ready to be a permanent spectator — at the stadium.

But not attending an Origin game for the first time — the series opener of 2007 at Suncorp — was tough. I knew, though, that it was the right decision not to go.

It was bang on three months after the operation (five days before my three-month check-up) and Gene Miles and some of the FOGS were very keen for me to attend; Geno was still trying to convince me up to the day of the game. But Jacqueline, in consultation with the medicos, was insistent that I didn't go.

Gene had invited me to watch the match from the FOGS' corporate area, where a seat alongside 'Tosser' Turner would have been guaranteed. While I would have been holed up away from the crowd in general, Jacqui believed that it would probably have increased the pressure I was under. As much as I really wanted to be at the match and initially challenged her views, after the game had passed I knew she was absolutely right. The former Origin players all congregate and have a drink before viewing the game and they get so passionate and vocal that, to an outsider, it must appear as though they're still playing from the comfort of the grandstand. I doubt I could have handled the excitement or fitted in very comfortably, considering the state of mind, and physical shape, I was in.

The traditional frenetic week-long countdown to the match was the toughest part to cope with. Plenty of journalists called to get my thoughts on the game, but Jacqueline politely told them I didn't want to give any opinion. I still didn't want to talk publicly and we knew the media couldn't have helped asking for a comment about my health. And, to be perfectly honest, I don't think I would have had too much to say about the match that was of any value anyway.

We had a group of family and friends come to our home to watch the game as Jacqueline probably believed that we needed some company to help me get through the frustration of not being there. Once the game started, my heart rate went through the roof; I could feel it pounding whenever Queensland scored and felt minor panic attacks when the Blues crossed.

I got so pumped up and agitated that, after about 15 minutes, I went out the back door and declared I was going to check the barbeque — even though it was an hour since I'd turned it off. The truth was that I had to get myself away to wind down a little, in case I brought a seizure on. After retirement, every time I watched a State of Origin match my heart pounded just like it used to prior to kick-off before any game I played.

I could still hear the cheers from inside the house and when I went back in to join the others, I had to keep telling myself not to get too excited. It would have been extremely ironic if an Origin match sparked a seizure, but thankfully the Maroons remained in control and eased my fears, winning 25–18. I can remember thinking, 'I'll struggle to get to sleep tonight,' but I was so comforted by the result I was completely at ease, even though I hadn't attended an Origin match for the first time in 27 years. A Maroons victory in State of Origin is the best medicine any Queenslander can receive.

It was a great victory for the Maroons, their third in a row after coming from 1–0 down to win the series the previous year, Mal Meninga's first as coach. It truly signified the emergence of a new era of Queensland players, the team going on to win that 2007 series and the next to make it three straight, the first time the mighty Maroons had done that since 1989.

As it turned out, I missed attending all three State of Origin games that 2007 season and watched them at home with the same group of people. However, some satisfaction came out of the final game of the series. Every year since it was struck in 2004, I would hand out a medal that carries my name, awarded to the player of the series; but in my absence, Mitchell was invited to make the presentation to the recipient, Queensland hooker Cameron Smith. It was a moment Mitch will never forget, and neither will I.

I was quickly realising that even though rugby league is the sport I have always loved so dearly, there are more important things in life. I had more time to spend with my family than I'd ever had before, and as my memory and energy improved I started to take more interest in other things. And I became more determined to play some sort of ambassador role for those who suffer epilepsy. I think I became less selfish, certainly less self-centred, and more aware of what was around me.

Ever so gradually, I began to become a little more self-confident in the ensuing months, even though I kept largely to the comfort of our home, and felt more assured about my chances for near complete recovery.

After my return home following surgery, Lane Calcutt had delivered a huge pile of letters addressed to me at Channel 9 that had arrived during my absence. But I was incapable of reading them. I just couldn't hold on to any slab of information for more than a few moments. That was evident every morning when I tried to read the newspaper; my long-time daily ritual became worthless. I'd start to read a story, but just a couple of lines in I'd have no idea of what it was about, and I'd return to the headline to gain a hint. That was a waste of time too, because my brain would have discarded the hint I'd just received from reading the story. So I gave up.

It was at about the six-month mark of my post-operative phase that my brain was working sufficiently to start reading again. So I grabbed that pile of letters and the number astounded me, as did where so many came from. As you would expect, there were plenty from Queenslanders but the number I received from throughout New South Wales was beyond belief. After representing Queensland for so long and being the most despised Maroons player during my career, I expected there wouldn't be too much support, let alone sympathy. But the messages of good wishes from south of the border, and the non-rugby league states, astounded me. There were 70 or 80 letters from Victoria, which I thought was perhaps because of my public praise for the Austin Medical Centre, but the numbers from Adelaide, Perth, Tasmania and the ACT countered that argument; plus I received a few from New Zealand, Papua New Guinea, and as far away as the United Kingdom. I was honestly overwhelmed and humbled by it.

There was one very special letter from Darwin, from Steve Shaw, who checked into the Austin that same day back in February 2007. He wished me all the best, as did his dad, and he updated me on how he was getting through his life with regular seizures, but remained buoyant as he always does. I knew that answering all these letters would take a while but I was determined to do it. I'd been warned about the difficulties that would arise out of having surgery on the left side of my brain, which would affect the right side of my body. I'm right handed, so I found using a biro a little tough. Writing wasn't a regular thing for me anyway; at work it's all about typing on a computer keyboard, which is far quicker than putting pen to paper. It wasn't until I was back at work that I tended to the replies, by hand, which I felt was more personal than by computer printout. But I also decided that, where possible and when I returned to an acceptable level of being able to communicate confidently, I'd provide a much more personal response to those who'd gone out of their way to think of me and telephone them to thank them personally.

Just as I placed the pile of letters down — it was late August — I received a call from Andrew Slack asking if it was okay to come over and visit. I told him he'd be very welcome and that there was also something I wanted to talk to him about. Typical of how my mind was then functioning, when he arrived and he asked me what that was, I'd completely forgotten — and to this day I have no idea what it was. That loss of memory process frustrated me so much.

Slacky asked me if returning to work was going to be a possibility at some stage. I'd shown him Dr O'Shea's staggered plan for my return, with a progressive increase in the hours and the days I could work. Slacky was comfortable with that, but he did say he wanted to take me to lunch one day before I returned to duty. It proved to be a double-bunger lunch rather than a double burger; not only did it include a tasty feed but also my first interview on camera since the operation, sitting alongside Broncos skipper Darren Lockyer. Basically the story was to unearth my opinions of Darren and talk about how important a captain's role can be. With Slacky in charge, I felt quite at ease during the interview, although I'm sure I didn't quite sound like the full quid.

The experience was a great confidence booster for me, and with the Channel 9 studios only a few kilometres from where we had lunch, Jacqueline and I decided to drop in and say hello to a few colleagues. It would only be a short visit of about 20 minutes but I was very nervous walking back into the place that I'd felt ashamed to leave months earlier. Yet everyone made me feel extremely welcome which I greatly appreciated. It was a little strange being back at my workplace though, not just because of the circumstances surrounding the last time I was there, but also because there'd been a bit of a shake-up in the television industry over the previous six months and there seemed to be very few people around compared to when I'd last been at the studios. Yet it was still wonderful to get to say 'g'day' to those who were there.

I think the only one who didn't enjoy the visit was news editor Ron Kruger. After he welcomed us back, Jacqueline thanked him for his help after my on-air drama and then fired a line at him: 'You men, you're all the same — you should be telling people about these problems.' Ron accepted the blame on my behalf.

I had to visit the Austin every three months for two years to check my progress. I was relieved when I received a better six-month report from the doctors at the Austin than I had three months prior. Although Professor Berkovic is never one to get too carried away, his assessment was: 'Yes, everything seems to be progressing as planned so far; see you next time.' That was enough to keep me happy. Marie O'Shea indicated that the return-to-work plan would be brought forward, although she demanded that it be followed with no alterations. She warned me that she'd seen many people get a little too confident too soon, and should that occur it could be back to the drawing board. Marie sent out a copy of my work schedule to Channel 9 station manager Lee Anderson and Andrew Slack with a note that her advice should be strictly adhered to.

My check-ups at the Austin Medical Centre would be conducted over two days — I'd go in for all the relevant scans to map my brain function. But the doctors advised that having a conversation with me almost told them as much about my progress as the advanced technology did. Dr O'Shea told me that they judged whether people were slow to respond to questions, hopeless at responding, whether the question would cause confusion or whether the person had improved so much that the response was regarded as quite fast. I used to try to judge how they were judging me, if I can put it that way. If I was slow at delivering an answer I'd get a little anxious. Usually it was a case of getting hit with one question after another as if the doctors were testing to see how quickly my brain could work.

I returned to Channel 9 in late September after an absence of almost 10 months, and my initial work schedule was just half a day on the Monday of the first week. To be honest, I don't think I lifted a finger but I went home and slept like a rock for 10 hours afterwards. My memory still wasn't real flash and I quickly discovered that even remembering a password for the computer was impossible. On the third day of coming in and having no idea how to log on with my password, I just wrote it down and stuck it on the side of the monitor — not particularly secure, but it was the only way I was going to be able to recall it. The next week my schedule increased to two half days a week and then three half days the next week. By the 10th week, I was back to five full days.

Fortunately, I was feeling physically and mentally strong enough by December 2007 to return to an annual charity golf event that I hated to miss — the Jack Newton Classic. I had been attending since the mid-1980s and the only one I've missed since was in 2006 — weeks after my on air-seizures. I'll always remember one of the first events I went to, in 1986. I flew in from the Kangaroo tour of England and France and Jacqui and the family met me at Brisbane airport. I gave my folks my touring bags, swapped them for a bag Jacqui had brought in with clothes for the weekend (and my golf clubs) and we headed straight up to Noosa to play at the Tewantin course. That's how keen I am to take part in Jack's event, where you get to mix and play with the cream of Australia's sport and entertainment talent, as well as plenty of political figures.

A real bonus during my return appearance in 2007 was that I got to meet one of my early music idols, Russell Morris, a bloke whose voice is just tremendous. I was lucky enough to see him perform, and it made my night to talk to him at Cypress Lakes.

During this period I returned to Melbourne and was relieved to receive another positive report. I'd just farewelled the office staff and was walking out of the epilepsy unit feeling very confident after nine months without a single seizure, when a woman came up to me and said, 'Would you mind coming over and seeing my son? He's very upset — he's just had a seizure.'

I walked over, introduced myself and started saying something like, 'It's a very important time of your life, and although considering having the surgery can make you a little bit nervous for a while, that can quickly disappear. It certainly did for me but, if you have the surgery then everything starts to change — life becomes much more fun again and ...'

At this point, the mother intervened. 'No no, I think you misunderstood me. My son has already had the surgery. He went nearly two years without a single seizure, he was just 10 days short of the two-year mark, actually, and then he had a major fit. Ten days short, that's all it was.'

The arse end fell out of me instantly. I couldn't believe it. The mother continued talking and, to be honest, I can't remember what she said after that. I was shattered. Why get so confident, I thought, after nine months, when in two years my seizures could return? Then I snapped out of it; it was important to continue with the mother's request to try to lift the spirits of her son. He was only 15, and I tried to console him the best I could. After a while, I asked him how regular his seizures were before he had the surgery. He replied, 'They were almost daily; if not, at least once every two days.' I could see how dejected he was, but I pointed out, 'Once every two years is a lot better than once every two days, isn't it?' He lifted his head for the first time and smiled. 'Yeah, I never thought of it that way; I'd rather have one every two years than every two days.'

It was good to leave him looking a lot brighter than when we were introduced, but to be honest it was something that plagued me for some time; my confidence levels took a pounding.

Shortly after that, I was approached by Madonna Williams — my son Lincoln's manager — to help with my affairs. Jacqueline had passed on any contact from the media to Madonna over the previous couple of months, and she thought it would be best that I did one exclusive

TV and one exclusive magazine interview to detail my battle with epilepsy — although I wasn't jumping out of my skin to do it. She asked what fee I'd request to do a story like that, as there'd been quite a bit of interest, with *60 Minutes*, *A Current Affair*, *Woman's Day*, *New Idea* and *The Courier Mail* all making inquiries. While I was happy for her to deal with all requests, I reminded her that, as I was still a Channel 9 employee, it could be difficult.

I'd been told that $30,000 was the normal fee paid for deals like this, but I wasn't sure, so I was content to leave it in Madonna's capable hands. A couple of weeks later she came to our place to deliver the news. 'How does 90 grand sound?' she smiled. I nearly fell off my seat. She'd bargained hard and that was the figure she'd been able to negotiate between *Woman's Day* and *A Current Affair*. Then it was time for me to surprise her when I declared that the money was to be donated to the Austin Medical Centre's epilepsy department and could she contact Sam Berkovic and ask him where to address the cheque (he allocated it to the Brain Research Centre). After Madonna calculated her commission and costs, which she'd certainly earned, I didn't keep one cent. It was a decision I was very content with.

Soon after, I did the *ACA* interview from my home in Brisbane with Amanda Paterson. The one thing I guaranteed them was that I wouldn't pull any punches; I'd tell the story as it was, even if the revelations were very embarrassing. And they were. The crew arrived and we went through the plans for the interview, digging into every detail, even the ones where I admitted to pissing my pants after suffering a seizure. I also detailed how I'd considered suicide, which was not something I was proud of. A stream of tears caused by bringing up the memory forced a bit of a delay.

The interview completed, I had to show the crew where on the pontoon I'd considered jumping off. Afterwards, I felt drained; but it was 'out there' and I just had to leave it in the producer's hands as far as how it was going to be portrayed.

It was three days short of a year since I'd had the surgery when *A Current Affair* screened the interview, on 18 February 2008. After I'd finished delivering the sports news, I walked into the news room and there didn't seem to be anyone in there. I continued a bit further and went past the boss's office; when I looked inside, it was chock-a-block full of people, maybe a dozen, all crowded around the monitors watching my interview. They were introducing the story at that stage, and quickly went to 'that fateful moment' on 30 November 2006 when I froze on screen. That was the first time I'd seen what had happened that night.

I stood at the side of the room. It was a bit surreal watching my confessions on the screen, and when it came to the part where I spoke about considering suicide, I felt a lump in my throat again. It was a bit awkward watching a crowd glued to the TV learning of my dilemma while I stood alongside them; I wouldn't say I felt embarrassed, but I was certainly anxious as I expected the shit was going to hit the fan with my workmates when they saw my candid confessions for the first time. At that stage I didn't know my admission that I'd pissed my pants on the set had been cut.

The segment screened for 18 minutes — including adverts — of the half-hour program (while there was another 12 minutes shown the following night). I slipped out the door before it had finished and I'd be subject to comment from everyone else, then waited for my mate from Nine and regular chauffeur Steve 'Spanner' Hopwood to finish his shift and give me a lift home.

The *ACA* interview was obviously the first point of discussion when I came in the door and, after not feeling all that comfortable with baring my soul on the television, Jacqui, Lincoln and Mitchell reassured me that they thought it came out fine, and my parents rang to say the same thing. Jacqui had been really worried about how my suicide thoughts would be played up, but it was included in the right context, and she was satisfied with how it came across. I slept well that night; I was relieved.

After being so private, even secretive, about my epilepsy for so long, it was a big thing to throw it all out there — but at least we were able to do it in one hit. *Woman's Day* hit the streets the next day and they ran a two-page spread. Although it had the headline 'Wally Lewis' secret depression battle: I WANTED TO END MY LIFE', it was less 'tabloid' in its angle than I expected. Jamie-Lee was visibly upset with the article, which seemed to centre upon my thoughts of suicide much more than my battle with epilepsy and the joys of overcoming the disease after surgery. Although she didn't let it out at home, she was very angry, and three days after struggling with the information, she broke down at school. She spoke with the house co-ordinator, who eased her tension greatly. From that day forward, Jamie-Lee seemed to have taken a closer interest in my daily health. Now fully aware of my condition, she even helped Jacqueline around the house … well for a little while, anyway.

The main thing I felt was relief — that my story was out, warts and all, and that the people I worked with knew my situation. But I was still only part of the way through my recovery and hadn't regained my confidence, so naturally there was some uneasiness there too.

A little while after I'd returned to work and started going out on jobs, a cameraman I regularly worked with, Paul Oliver, asked how I was feeling and said that he thought my scar had healed really well. 'Ollie' had a scar on his forehead, but I didn't know how he'd got it — I thought it could have been in a car accident or some other way; it wasn't really my business. One day he told me that, quite a few years earlier, he too had had major brain surgery for epilepsy, and that his scar hadn't healed as well as mine had. We became closer and I found quite a bit of comfort in knowing that he'd had the surgery and made a good recovery, having had no seizures since his operation.

Progressively, I started to feel myself again. The first six months had been horrendous — I'd really felt like I was five cents short in the dollar when it came to mental capacity — but I could certainly notice a big step forward between my six-month and 12-month check-ups. However, my lack of memory was still worrying me badly. It was a very, very slow recovery, but then again I was probably a little impatient too. Before having the operation, I was warned by Professor Berkovic that my memory might never be great again and that I shouldn't get frustrated by it. It has certainly improved quite a bit now, though, since those first few months after the surgery.

I was still suffering a bit of depression but nothing like what it had been. Being back at Channel 9 assisted that — I always had plenty of company, and great support from my colleagues. My concern about not being able to remember small things still rattled me; sometimes I'd have to go back in to check the list of my assigned stories, or occasionally I'd complete my stories only to be told I'd forgotten something. Slacky was wonderful — he'd say, 'What does it matter? Don't get too upset.' One good thing now is that at least my memory can be prompted if I forget something; it's not lost forever. Someone will say something to me and I'll think, 'That's right,' and it will come back to me, whereas previously there was just nothing there. At the 12-month mark I could really sense within myself I was remembering quite a few more things.

Socially I was still very nervous and stand-offish, particularly with people I hadn't met before. I wouldn't make the first move to talk and it took a while to shake that, but the doctors kept reiterating that it was just a natural lack of confidence and in time it would return.

It's fascinating what the surgery did to certain characteristics I had. Other than my sudden taste for tea and distaste for coffee, I also used to love seafood but suddenly I wasn't very partial to it at all. I've always liked my steaks well done, almost burnt, but took to liking them being medium rare. Jacqui noticed that, for some time, if someone dropped a spoon or made an unexpected noise, I would turn around a bit startled, whereas previously I wouldn't have even noticed. I'm not one to feel the cold, and in the middle of winter, while Jacqui would be freezing and have the rugs pulled up to her ears in bed, I'd sleep on top of the sheet and only pull it over me if I felt a little chilly. After the operation I was tucked up under the covers feeling really cold; even when I sat on the lounge I'd have a blanket over me.

Jacqui knew I was getting better when I didn't need the sheet over me any more and dropped off drinking so much tea. Now I'm back to three or four coffees a day — but it took over two years.

Fortunately, I'm on far less medication than before but I still have no urge to drink alcohol; I've been off it so long I'm quite happy with continuing and Jacqui doesn't drink either. My abstinence goes back to the days when I was working for the beer brands, when I was always conscious of what a public relations disaster it would be for them and for me if I was ever caught drink driving or just drunk in public, so I curbed my intake then; but also, it was never wise to overindulge anyway with the amount of medication I consumed over many years.

Bit by bit, the pieces were coming together. Yet I was still apprehensive about going back in front of the camera to read the sports news. Inevitably, I knew I had to resume the role at some stage. And when I did, my fear raised itself all over again.

ANOTHER PERSPECTIVE

By Ken Brown, Coast Watch *celebrity*

In the first few weeks after Wally returned from his operation in Melbourne, our great mate 'Tosser' Turner appointed me to make sure Wally was okay. Living in the next suburb and having tried to allay any fears he had about the surgery before going under the knife, it was a role I was happy to play.

As mates often do when the chips are down, I tried to make light of the situation. And I'd report my observations of Wally's progress to Tosser while regularly getting advice from Pete Silburn, the neurologist who had organised the operation.

When Pete told me the time was right, I lobbed around to Wally's for a visit and we spent a couple of hours talking about State of Origin games and players from the late-'80s and early-'90s. Wally didn't realise at the time that old 'Brownie' was following Pete Silburn's advice to get him to talk about the past. Pete had warned me that Wally's short-term memory would be rat-shit, but that his long-term memory wouldn't be too bad, so I steered the conversation that way.

The next big step was for him to leave the house and go somewhere without Jacqui. The plan was to do something simple the first time, so I picked him up and took him for a drive along the Wynnum and Manly foreshores and to have lunch at my house.

When I arrived to pick him up, Wally got in the car but realised he'd forgotten his sunglasses. He went back in the house to get them but forgot what he was doing there. This happened four times and he started to become distressed. I tried to soften the moment. 'Is that all … that's nothing … happens to me all the time … and I never got hit in the head like you.'

Wal arrived at our place to see our little dog Rufus, who, unbeknown to Wally, had been having seizures and was a suspected epileptic. My wife Shelly and I had arranged with our vet to rush the little bloke there next time he had a seizure, so they could take a blood sample and ascertain for sure what the problem was.

Wally had just settled on the lounge and Rufus came over wagging his tail. Wally gave him a pat and Rufus' left leg went out at 90 degrees to his body, and he began to shake and fell over right in front of him. I jumped up and called Shelly to grab the dog and rush him to the vet. I then looked at Wal and said with a big grin on my face, 'Stuff you, King ... you've come around to my house and given my dog epilepsy!'

I ran off to phone the vet to let him know the dog was on the way. When I returned to the room Wally was on the phone to Jacqui telling her there was a crisis at Brownie's and maybe she should pick him up. He was rocking gently back and forward in the seat, tears streaming down his face. I thought I'd upset his fragile mental state and started to feel guilty. I said, 'Oh geez, Wal ... I'm sorry, mate ... I was only kiddin' about you giving my dog "eppo". I didn't mean it, mate ... are you alright?'

Wally smiled back at me. 'Listen, you idiot, I'm not upset ... these are tears of laughter. And it's the first time I've had a good laugh since before the operation.'

Shortly after that episode, I drove the King up to Sandgate to have lunch at the Fish Co-Op with Tosser and his wife Jan. Toss arranged for Geno [Gene

Miles] and Badge [Gary Belcher] to drop by and say hello before lunch, and it was a good day spent in the company of good friends. On the way home, as we cruised over the Gateway Bridge, a plumber's truck with a couple of likely looking lads in it cruised up in the lane beside us and they gave the King a wave.

Wal looked at the sign on the side of the truck which said 'Your Shit Is Our Business' and immediately cracked up laughing; although he was a bit worried the blokes thought he was laughing at them for waving, and not the sign.

Making humour despite Wally's situation was important during the two-year period while he waited to see if the operation was a success. Three months before the two years was up, I called him and asked if he wanted to do a test run on his health and take advantage of fourth-row seats I had for the John Mellencamp and Sheryl Crow concert. 'There's nothing like flashing lights and loud music when it comes to sending an epileptic off ... so do you want to come and see if you can handle it?' I asked him.

He and Jacqui had a great night, although I had a scary moment early in the concert when I thought he might have been having a seizure; only to realise it was his unco-ordinated way of moving to the music. Tragic! It was so good to see people saying hello and wishing him well that night; nice to see him back doing things he'd avoided for years.

Epilepsy is a serious condition and Wally was coming out of a hellish period, so I don't mean to make light of that at all. But mates' humour is often the best tonic in tough situations and I'm sure Wally appreciated me and others taking the piss out of him as he slowly regained his old character after the operation. It was so good to see him laugh, and eventually fire back insults sharply as if the menace was back in his make-up.

The King is back.

FIFTEEN

BACK ON THE BIKE

A S MY work hours increased, so did my confidence back in front of the camera. Physically and mentally I was feeling more and more at ease turning up for work each day at Channel 9 ... until I had to get 'back on the bicycle'.

I was told I'd return to the news desk to read the sport 'at some stage'; the longer it went before any detail was added to 'that day', the more comfortable I felt. I was so tentative that several times I deflected inquiries from management asking when I thought I'd be ready to go back onto the desk, and I even put off a couple of planned return dates. Lee Anderson assured me my return would be done 'discreetly', with no big build-up. I remember asking him if he was going to promote the fact that I was returning to reading the sports news and, if so, to let me know when the promos would start so I could make sure

I didn't turn the TV on. I wanted to stay away from the pressure or any expectations that would be built up. Finally, Lee confirmed I'd be going back to the front line 'sometime next week' and assured me it would be a 'low-key return'. But I was still petrified.

It was decided that Steve Haddan, who'd read the news most nights in my absence, would be scheduled to do the job on this particular night. I'd come onto the set and sit next to him and he'd officially welcome me back.

When the night came I could feel the heart pounding, and I was constantly questioning whether I could feel any light palpitations of the heart. The thoughts kept rushing through my mind: 'Am I feeling light tingles? Am I going to screw up again?'

Steve and I had known each other for over 20 years, and having him there to ease me in helped make my return easier. Once we were on air, he welcomed me back to the news desk, asked me a few questions about rugby league and had a brief conversation, mentioning that I'd return to the job in the next few nights. Steve then read the sports news and I took a back seat.

Two nights later, I was back on the bike. Bruce Paige and Heather Foord were obviously on a mission to relieve the pressure; and it worked. I'd been suffering fits for almost 30 years but, this particular night, I was thrust into a different fit altogether; a fit of laughter. When the tape was rolling of news items, as well as during the ad breaks, they were talking their heads off with stupid gibber and wisecracks — obviously trying to take my mind off my fear of a disastrous return. Despite the pressure I felt, I couldn't help but smile.

And then I heard those familiar, once fearful, words in my earpiece: '*Ten seconds, Wal ...*'

The nerves were jangling.

'*Five ... four ... three ... two ... one.*'

Before I began to preview the upcoming sport, Bruce Paige welcomed me back to the desk after my long absence. I looked at the camera and thanked, from my heart, all the Channel 9 viewers and sports fans from around the country who'd made my recovery a little easier. I felt very comfortable doing that, but less comfortable coming back after the commercial break to read the sports news.

The five or six commercials seemed to pass by in an instant, and suddenly I was back on the screen, looking directly at the camera.

As I began reading my first story, I could feel my voice breaking up. With a hint of a nervous quiver, it was like I was addressing an audience at high school for the first time. I'm sure it sounded terrible but my biggest concern was not the inflection or the conviction of my voice, but getting through without a seizure. I felt unbelievably relieved when I'd finished. Confidence is a wonderful thing; it grew sentence by sentence that night.

Following my exit from the newsroom, everyone around me told me how good I was; even though I suspect some of the well wishers hadn't even seen me on screen. But I appreciated their efforts to instill a bit of confidence in me.

I didn't hang around the station too long at all; I briefly saw Lee and Slacky and left hurriedly. Jacqui was waiting outside in the car: she'd wanted to come into the studio to provide a little support, but couldn't bring herself to; she was feeling the tension as much as I was. When I reached the car, there was a massive pressure release. Jacqueline got halfway through asking if I was okay before bursting into tears; then again, I might have beat her to it. Here we were, both blubbering in the car as the emotion and the relief just flooded out of me.

When I arrived home the kids were great and I received a couple of phone calls of support which ensured I slept well; very well. A first major hurdle had been navigated. I certainly can't remember being that nervous or uncertain about myself when I debuted for Valleys, Queensland or Australia. However, life was very different then.

From that night, bit by bit over the next few months, I felt more relaxed on the news desk and more assured that the seizures were behind me. I could prepare for reading the news each night without having to be on-guard for a sudden surge through my body, and it's hard to put into words the feeling of being able to do my job without terror constantly being just half a step behind me.

The support and loyalty I received from the Channel 9 management is something I appreciated so much. My contract (and I'd assume that any standard television contract would be the same) stipulated that if I couldn't perform my duties for three months in any 12-month period, my services could be terminated. And given that my contract expired at the end of 2007, I was naturally concerned about my career, and financial future, while I was laid up recovering at home.

In May 2007, three months after the operation, my good friends Ken Brown and Dick Turner met with Lee Anderson to seek clarification of my contractual situation on my behalf and Lee was nothing but supportive and reassuring that he wanted me to remain at Channel 9 long term. The television industry was going through a tough economic time and there had been a lot of pruning of staff and changes at high levels, so as a show of loyalty it was tremendous. I have since renewed my contract again, which will extend my time at Channel 9 for another couple of years.

The 12-month anniversary of my surgery arrived in February 2008 and I returned to Melbourne for my check-up. Once again the event was covered by Lane Calcutt for Nine and he got a shot of me greeting Sam Berkovic and Gavin Fabinyi. Before the camera went on, I approached Sam and Gavin and said I wanted to privately thank them for making my life fun again. I seemed to stun them a little but I was serious, and sincere. The cameras then started rolling as I provided a public thank you to them, and presented the cheque for $75,000 (my net income, after agency costs and commission, from the *ACA/Woman's Day* interviews — I didn't keep one cent).

After that was all over, I walked into a couple of rooms to say hello to some patients. It was a trip down memory lane for me; I took a look at the room I'd been in a year earlier and recalled my days in the chair beneath the overhead camera, and the times I spent praying for seizures rather than fearing them. I visited a lovely young girl whose mother was quite keen to talk about how she was struggling to overcome the discomfort of being hooked up to machines and to face what lay ahead as she went through the same monotonous routine I'd had to endure. Her mother gave us permission to get a shot of the girl lying there as I entered the room to talk to her. Just as I entered, the cameras trailing me, she had a massive seizure. Nurses rushed to her room and the alarms were sounding. It was a terrible moment to experience.

Surprisingly, her mother came out and approached us half an hour later, just before we left the hospital. She said her daughter would like to have us back inside. I think it was Mum's idea, though; the girl seemed a little uncomfortable and I insisted that, if she felt embarrassed in the least, to just say no to the cameras capturing her. She gave us the green light and quickly settled down. She was a brave young lady. The footage went to air a couple of days later, and the telling of her story increased the awareness of epilepsy and the battles for those who suffer it.

Despite plenty of coverage over the years, it appears that the big 'e' confuses millions of people around the country, including those who suffer from it and their families. While I've been a keen promoter of rugby league and breweries over the years, most of my comments have now changed to assisting those suffering the disease. It's the least I can do after all the support from the medical experts, family, friends and the many people I have never met, who gave me such good wishes.

As part of my 12-monthly analysis from the doctors,

again I received the 'so far, so good' comment. During these two-day stays, which were three months apart, they'd do extensive testing of my progress. I'd have a series of scans which would monitor my brain activity and check how the part of the brain affected by the surgery was functioning.

I also did some physical tests during my three- and six-month check-ups, as I hadn't done anything more demanding in that time than work around the back yard. I brought up the subject of my eye sight as I'd been warned that this type of surgery could cause trouble with the eyes. Other than staring at the box most of the day, I was hardly exercising them, and I hadn't been reading because it was a bit too testing for me. But I was told my eyes were fine.

The fact I'd gone a year without a seizure pleased the medical team, but for me it also beckoned a new chapter in my life — I could drive a car again. Any patient who undergoes the brain surgery has to be seizure-free for a full year and have a medical clearance before a driving licence can be re-issued (for only 12 months at a time), and I was very keen to get that bit of freedom back. I had taken to catching the train to work most days; on the others, Jacqui would drive me in and I'd either get the train back or get a lift with Steve Hopgood.

As I've mentioned, Andrew Slack has been a tower of strength, giving me great support. But being a boss, he also knew he had to push me along. It was well beyond a year after my surgery that I started to really gather some confidence. That was due to a lot of help from people around me and the work schedule that Slacky gave me which kept me occupied; although the weekend shift was hard to get used to at first. I read the news on Friday, Saturday and Sunday nights, and compiled stories on Thursday and Monday nights relating to the weekend matches. Saturdays also included doing reviews of the two Friday night games and also providing live progress of the early Saturday game; while on Sundays I'd do the wrap-ups of that day's action, as well as the two late games played on Saturday night. It helped that I was talking about rugby league, the sport I love so much.

Lee Anderson called me aside one day and said he'd had a request from Sydney for me to join the State of Origin commentary team for the 2008 series. He told me it was up to me, but the station obviously felt that if I was confident enough to read the news live, being at the footy with a heap of other Nine commentators would be less stressful.

Being shifted from the Origin panel years earlier was one of the things that had disappointed me the most during my

TV career; it was the arena I felt most suited to and comfortable in, but I'd written off ever returning. The Sydney crew had Peter Sterling, Paul Vautin, Phil Gould, Paul Harragon, the Johns brothers, then Steve Walters and Ben Ikin from Brisbane — and I think Gary Belcher at one time.

When I thought about Lee's proposal, it was an opportunity to work closer to the game by being part of Origin night again, and I felt I would have been mad not to give it a go. But I was petrified that first night: I was happy the shots were of my waist upwards only, so the viewers didn't see my knees rattling. I was thinking, 'What if I stuff up? What if pressure and nerves cause me to have a seizure here?' Once I spoke the first two or three times I felt more relaxed. That fear elapsed but it was quickly replaced by another fear — of saying something stupid and making myself look like a numbskull. However, after the second game I felt much better and by the third, I felt like I belonged there again.

A few weeks before the 2008 State of Origin series began, there was one more memorable trip to Melbourne, in early May, that will always be a significant part of the Lewis' family history, and this time the destination wasn't the Austin Medical Centre.

Lincoln had been nominated as a finalist in one of the categories at the Logie Awards, and of course it was an event not to be missed. Jacqueline's sister Kayleen and her two kids Dean and Carla joined Jacqui, Mitchell, Jamie-Lee and me and headed down for the big night.

Unfortunately, we hadn't been invited to the Logies presentations, so we booked into a hotel not far away from the event, so the kids could get a glimpse of the stars as they made their way into the function. I was pretty keen to grab a feed straight after the red carpet activities but the girls wanted to make sure we returned to the room in time to guarantee we didn't miss anything. That meant ordering a couple of delivered pizzas — even though we still had another hour and a half until the telecast began!

And didn't the tension increase dramatically as the program came on the television! After a couple of awards were presented, the blood pressure around the room seemed to increase, and then my mobile phone went off. It was a message from Fatty Vautin, and just as I began to read it Jacqueline's mobile also rang. Fatty's message said, 'Congratulations. Your son has just won a Logie for the best new talent.' My first thought was, 'Fatty's trying to gee me up again.' We had dropped a couple of shockers on each other over the years, but I thought to myself, 'Surely he couldn't hit me with bullshit as personal as this … could he?'

Then Jacqueline confirmed the news. Her call, from Lincoln's agent Madonna Williams, informed us that it was indeed true but our celebrations didn't really get underway until we'd seen the actual announcement ourselves, half an hour later on the delayed telecast.

Eventually we headed down to the post-presentation function to catch up, and after Jacqueline finally stopped impersonating 'Woody Woodpecker' by monotonously kissing Lincoln's cheek, I got a chance to congratulate him myself. Mitchell smiled and came out with the line that his brother would be referred to differently from now on; no longer was Linc to be called Wally Lewis' son, but I'd be tagged 'Lincoln Lewis' father'. It was a very proud night for all of us.

Once again, I'd experienced plenty of emotion in Melbourne, but there wasn't one thought about having a seizure.

Also in 2008, I returned to public speaking for the first time for nearly two years, at LJ Hooker's annual national sales awards at the Tattersall's Club in Brisbane. I got up in front of quite a few hundred people, received some nice applause, thanked the organisers for the invitation and said something along the lines of, 'There's only one thing I ask you to understand — that I'm going to be nervous, as this is the first time I've spoken in public since I've had brain surgery.' The Queensland manager pounced on this a bit with, 'Ah, *this* is *the* first time, eh, at an LJ Hooker function.' Anyway, I continued, 'If I make a bit of a fool of myself — if I start speaking Egyptian, Swahili, or upside down — just remember that part of my brain is missing and obviously the surgery didn't work as well as I would have thought. But at least my illness is now out there and you know about it.'

I received a few nervous giggles and polite applause and then went on to be interviewed about rugby league and epilepsy before presenting the awards. I'm sure those closest to the stage could see my arms and legs shaking, and my thumbs and fingers fidgeting as I spoke: the ultimate 'no no' for anyone in the TV industry. At the end, I felt I'd made a real step forward in my recovery. I'd told the organisers before the luncheon I was very happy to sign things, have photographs taken with people and chat with their guests, but I had to go to another commitment shortly after the awards had been made. So I departed early, and as soon as I sat in my car I just let out a big gasp and sat for a few seconds as if a huge pressure had been released from my body.

I took on one or two more speaking engagements and charity functions after that and week by week I started to feel more comfortable back in front of the camera or microphone. Lee Anderson gave me a progress report just recently when he told me he thought I was going along 'okay' and seemed to have got a lot more confidence back, then added the dreaded 'but …'.

He spoke about the need for me to relax more when presenting the sports news, and read more like I would in a conversation with my mates, without too much emphasis in my delivery. I laughed at what a colleague at Channel 10 had told me when I first started in the industry 20 years earlier; to drum up my delivery, with a lot more emphasis and animation in certain parts of the sentence. When I said, 'But I don't talk like that,' he told me that if I wanted a future in television, I'd better learn. Now I had someone telling me the opposite; it shows how times have changed.

Talking about times changing, Lane Calcutt walked past me one day and targeted a cutting insult at me. But I was on my game and snapped back with a sharp response. He stopped for a second and commented, 'You *must* be better, King; this has started all over again!' There were definitely some things I'd missed while being away from Channel 9, and insulting him in our daily exchanges was one of them.

Now we can't walk past without bagging the hell out of each other. It's good to be back.

ANOTHER PERSPECTIVE

By Steve Crawley, Channel 9 head of sport

I'll never forget that night. It was mid-2003 and I was producing my first State of Origin series for Channel 9. We were at Suncorp Stadium, and in the distance eating his dinner, alone, stood 'The King'.

Our outside broadcast trucks set up in the bowels of the stadium and dinner is served on plastic plates with food to match. But it's a long night and it's best to get something down before the big game. Nine's crew on Origin nights number north of 100 people, and we eat in a massive happy huddle.

Except for Wally. He'd just hosted the sports news for QTQ9 Brisbane out on the field but was not part of the actual Origin coverage. Can you believe that? We couldn't find an on-camera role for the biggest legend in the history of the series.

It took me two, maybe three minutes to ask, '*Why?*' 'Well,' said one of the senior staff, 'poor old Wally's off with the pixies. You'll get him on a panel, he'll go off on a tangent and you can't stop him ...'

Bugger that. So we got Wally on the panel at the very next Origin, alongside 'Sterlo' and 'Fatty', and guess what? He began brilliantly before going off on a tangent and we couldn't stop him. Sure, we had a problem but Wally had a bigger one, even though back then he wouldn't admit it to anyone, including himself.

Since his operations and recovery, he's become an invaluable member of Nine's rugby league coverage; not just Origins but everything from *Friday Night Football* to grand finals and Test matches.

Fast forward ...

We were in Melbourne for a match during the 2008 World Cup, waiting outside our hotel for a ride to the ground, when I told Wally how great he was going, how different it was compared to a couple of years back when everyone literally held their breaths whenever he went on air.

'You don't know what a relief it is,' he said; quietly though, through that crooked smile of his. 'Back then, I'd be walking along at the football and I'd piss my pants. Had no control ... I'd have to keep walking as if nothing had happened. It was bloody hard.'

Just to get back to where he is now, Wally Lewis is a bigger hero than any of us ever knew. We should all be happy for him and at the same time appreciate him for exactly what he is — a champion.

SIXTEEN

BY HIS SIDE

By Jacqueline Lewis

IT is just so wonderful to have the real Wally Lewis back in my life: the strong, invincible 'I can do anything' type of man that I married. He was gone for a long while.

In fact, Wally is a better man now, I believe, because of what he has gone through. He is more conscious of others, more compassionate, patient, tolerant, and he even shows real emotion sometimes!

I know it will seem a bit strange that I say this, but I'm glad he had a seizure while on air at Channel 9, because it took that embarrassing experience for him to finally confront his epilepsy and do something about it; which led down the path of the operation that has changed our lives. It took that to shake him into action.

When everything came to a head at the end of 2006, I'd been at him for a while to let go of the secret; but I'd almost given up hope that he would. When he had the first on-air seizure two weeks earlier, I tried so hard to convince him to end the charade. I told him, 'You've got to come out, because this is crazy. People are making up their own scenarios — like you've had a minor stroke on TV or were drunk.' That didn't seem to worry him but I just thought he had to acknowledge what was wrong with him and face it head on, because I was sick of the fear and worry.

A seizure happening on screen wasn't a matter of 'if', but 'when'. I could see he was getting worse in the months beforehand; he was having seizures more regularly and was always very tired. I knew in my heart that it was heading to a really bad place.

While Wally's biggest fear was having a seizure in front of the cameras, mine was him having one behind the wheel of the car, especially during the last five years before the operation, as I could see him deteriorating more and more as time went on; he'd be sitting at home regularly having seizures and just riding them out.

I was most scared when Wally was driving home after work — I'd count the minutes until he walked in the door. I'd be worried he might have a turn and go over the edge coming down Mount Coot-tha. I knew what time he should be home from work and I'd be watching the clock, thinking, 'Why is he not here?' Often he'd ring me when he might be 10 or 20 minutes from being home, asking whether I wanted anything picked up; if he was late and hadn't rung, I'd start to panic.

I became the driver, the kids' chauffeur, and I enjoyed it to be honest. I couldn't ask Wally to go pick them up from a party or night club. He never did any of that because I couldn't have him driving in the middle of the night, endangering not only his own life, but others'.

Now if I have to pick up Jamie-Lee at the airport if she's coming in from interstate late, Wally will say, 'I'll come.' When we're at the airport talking to other parents while waiting for the girls, it's like, 'Oh my God, I've got a husband.' Others used to say to me, 'Why do you always pick her up?' In other words, 'Why doesn't Wally share the load?' But I had to take on that responsibility. It's nice now when he says, 'I'll come with you to pick the kids up,' or 'I'll go and pick them up, you stay there; you stay asleep.' Wow!

Wally's epilepsy has been part of our lives since I was pregnant with Lincoln. We had no idea what epilepsy was really about. It was like finding out Jamie-Lee was profoundly deaf. It was a real shock but we learned and we searched everywhere we could and we were determined to leave no stone unturned. We thought: we'll get communication for her, we'll never give up and we'll communicate with our wonderful daughter one day. I should have gone and learned a lot more about epilepsy as well, so I could understand it better, and I regret that now, but I was so pre-occupied doing all I could for our daughter that I overlooked how vulnerable my husband had become.

The seizures had gradually got more frequent and worse. Wally documents the awful one he had in front of me when we were at the Gold Coast, which was frightening. I admit I would 'lose it' sometimes if he had a seizure when I was there; and I used to fear what would happen if the boys or I weren't around, as somebody else mightn't even know he was having one. In time, we learned to deal with them.

At first, Wally was able to live quite well and just ride out the seizures but he slowly became more withdrawn and unconfident. The Wally I met and fell in love with was strong, almost invincible; he knew exactly what he was doing and wanted to achieve. You had a sense that nothing was going to get in his way or hold him back. Wally was also very passionate about his country and his game: it was his first love, I accepted that.

Gradually he became reclusive. He was slowly losing himself. I tried to hide things from him that might worry him or upset him and trigger a seizure. As the epilepsy held him back, suddenly there were doubts within the make-up of the great Wally Lewis that became obvious. I learned how dreadful it must be for anyone suffering epilepsy. Wally knew what he wanted to do or say but he'd have a seizure and it would come out differently or he'd lose concentration or not remember things, and he had such a good memory. It put him on edge, not knowing when those things would happen.

And he knew he was dodging bullets every time he had to do something live on camera, and it's probably amazing to think he only got caught out four times.

The one I felt worst about was when he had a seizure while filming *This Is Your Life* in 2002. I blame myself for that; I should have said he couldn't do it when the producers approached me. I knew that was going to be an uncomfortable situation for him and he'd been really busy and really tired recently, which made the likelihood of having a seizure greater. But because no one knew about his epilepsy and how it affected him, it was hard to come up with a reason to avoid the show.

I knew exactly what was going on while he stumbled on his words that day, and I felt so helpless not being able to help him. He was really bad that night after the show; very drained. He went to bed when we got home and didn't talk. I felt very ill. I felt like I should have said no

— that, knowing his fear, I shouldn't have exposed him to that happening.

After the *This Is Your Life* program and his seizure the year before while reading the sports news, I wanted Wally to explain his epilepsy to the public. People were whispering about him and guessing what had happened. I thought, 'This is wrong — you need to have people aware of the truth.' About that time there were a couple of speaking engagements he did with Mark Ella and he was up on stage and had mild seizures and stumbled with his talking. I heard some bloke behind me say one time, 'He's had a few too many,' and ridiculed him. I thought, 'You have no idea.' But it was no use defending him in front of people like that, because they didn't know what was really happening. I felt then he should have come out and acknowledged it; but in saying that, the media often sensationalise things and, before you know it, it becomes the subject of ridicule rather than something serious.

A few months before he had his two seizures on air in 2006, our great friend Dick Turner — God rest his beautiful soul — could tell Wally was struggling. He said to me, 'We're losing him. We have to get Wally out of TV; it's too much pressure on him.' He started talking about some other possible career opportunities for Wally.

By that stage there were many things Wally didn't attend, because he no longer felt comfortable being in the public eye and I'd always make an excuse; he was busy or had other commitments. The truth was that often he'd be at home asleep. Even at Christmas, we'd start to play cricket at his brother's place and Wally would leave early, and go home to rest. The good thing was that our families knew about his epilepsy so he didn't have to make any excuse.

Throughout his career — whether it was when he played or trained, or was at work — he'd given every bit of energy he had, and when he got home, he often had nothing more to give.

I'm a talker, as anyone who knows me will tell you. I love communication, but with Wally he'd come home and not want to talk, and that was very hard. Now we talk; we can have an argument without me fearing I've upset him and maybe put him in a position where he might have a seizure. Now I can 'get up' him for not putting the garbage bin out, whereas before I'd do it, not wanting to disturb him, or he might be asleep on the lounge chair and I didn't want to wake him.

He missed doing things with the kids. Even when they had their friends over, he'd often go to another room and just sit there because he was so tired. That's all changed now. I'll never forget a night a few months ago when Lincoln had some of the cast from *Home and Away* stay over. Wally was out the back talking and laughing with them and I couldn't stay up and keep pace with them, so I excused myself and went to bed. Mitchell and Lincoln have embraced that so much now; they love having their dad mix with their friends. Even when Wally couldn't drive and Lincoln and Mitchell had to chauffeur him around, Lincoln told me he thought it was great because 'we get to hang out'. It's been a bit harder for Jamie-Lee — I don't think she's quite as comfortable with her father being a chatterbox with other parents when she's wanting to be taken home!

The first two times Wally had seizures while presenting the Channel 9 sport were when I was away and he was tired and run down from the break in routine. In 2001, I was in the USA with Mitchell after taking him to a camp in Alabama, learning about the space missions. We got home on the Sunday and Wally insisted that he meet us at the airport, which was really silly because I knew it would make him tired after all the travelling he'd been doing covering games for Fox Sports. But he hadn't seen us for 18 days, so he met us early in the morning, before having to get on another plane a few hours later and then getting home late that night. The next night he had a seizure on air.

Then, when he had his first of the two in November 2006, I'd been away with Jamie-Lee for a water polo championships and he just seemed to get run down and really tired. Sure enough, he had a seizure while reading the news.

I always tried to watch him do the news every night, whether at home or on a small battery-powered TV I'd take with me. Mitchell would always try to watch his father too: not to see what he had to say — it was more hold his breath and make sure Dad got through it okay.

When Wally had the second seizure in front of the camera that November, I started crying and screaming, 'This can't be happening — not again!' Mitchell was supposed to have gone out but, again, he'd waited until his father got through reading the news first, as one of us always did.

We had family at our place — everyone was in a panic — and I sent Mitchell and Lincoln in to pick Wally up. Jamie-Lee was 16 then and she knew nothing about Wally's epilepsy; we felt she had enough issues and didn't need to be burdened with her father's problems. I knew, though, that I finally had to tell her what was going on: she needed to know the full extent of this situation. She got very defensive when we explained everything to her and asked why we hadn't told her before then. She thought it was unfair that she hadn't known while Lincoln and Mitchell had.

The boys have been absolutely terrific all these years. They used to keep an eye on Wally all the time and were used to coming up with reasons why he couldn't attend this or that. I would have the boys on alert. They are like rocks; they were constantly there to make sure their father was okay. They took on a big responsibility. Mitchell was always making sure he was watching his father and to make sure Dad got through a seizure, if he was aware he was having one. They were good minders. From the age of about seven, Mitchell knew it was an issue but in his teens he became more aware. Lincoln has always looked up to Mitchell and been guided by him, so if Mitchell said, 'We're looking after Dad,' he would never question it.

I'll never forget being in Noel Saines' office the day after Wally's last on-air seizure when I learned they'd been talking about the option of surgery since 2004, and that Noel had suggested Wally consider the move. Wally had only told me the night before that Noel had again mentioned surgery; however, Noel assumed I'd been told about it after their original conversation.

On the way home from that visit I told Wally I wanted to give Peter Silburn a call to get a second opinion, and Peter was great in arranging for us to go in after his office had closed one evening, so there'd be no one around. Seeing him was the best decision we made.

Peter said afterwards that Wally was having mini-seizures while they were speaking but didn't realise it; that his brain would have got so used to them that he wouldn't really be aware of them. Normally when a patient is on three lots of medication, they look at having the operation: Wally was on four. Peter told him, 'It's amazing you're not permanently asleep on this medication.' He was always tired but most other people wouldn't have handled that dosage.

It was up to Wally to decide if he had the surgery. There are always some dangers with major surgery, and he was the one suffering and knew what he needed to do. It was different with Jamie-Lee; our responsibility was to make that decision for her. My biggest fear in the surgery was getting him out alive; from then on I knew we could get through it. Post-op can be very tough — we went through that twice with Jamie-Lee, so to a degree we knew what to expect.

Since Wally's plight was revealed, the support we've received from so many people, from close friends to strangers, has just been overwhelming. That is so special to us and I can't thank people enough.

But it wasn't enough for Wally during his post-operation

period when he was so terribly hit with depression. I thank God that Penny Kincade rang our number one day when I was out picking up the kids and she spoke to Wally. Any other time she rang, I was there to answer the phone and she would check Wally's progress through me. But this time she spoke to Wally and he let her know how depressed he was. She called back after I got home, and she said, 'Jacqui, I need to talk to you; we need to talk about Wally getting some anti-depressant medication.' I said, 'Oh no, Penny, he's fine. I know about it [depression]. I told you about my brother John's battle. I know Wally's not very well at the moment, but we'll get him there. I know he's going through a little bit of a hurdle.'

She said, 'No, Jacqui, that's a different depression — this is a chemical imbalance sparked by what happened to Wally during his operation. This is different, okay? I've just got off the phone from Wally and he's in a bad place.'

I was thinking, 'No, not more medication.' I thought an extra cuddle or an 'I love you' would be enough. This is Wally, this isn't my baby brother John, who just couldn't get out of his deep hole, no matter what we did or said. No, Wally is not that bad, I thought. He'll be fine.

But I started to think hard about what Penny had said. Early next morning, while the kids were asleep, I went to buy some milk, telling Wally I'd only be gone 10 minutes.

While I was out, I ran into a friend who also suffers epilepsy, and we started talking. Before I realised it, I'd been gone 20 minutes and rushed home. At the time, I just never left him very often and wherever I went in the house he was behind me, like my dog. When I came back from the shops he was sitting there at the kitchen bench — he hadn't moved an inch; hadn't even turned the TV on. He was just sitting, staring into space. I thought, 'Okay, you're in a bad place and it's out of my control; a hug or an "I love you" isn't going to make it better.'

So Wally took the medication and we could see the improvement in him quickly; but he still did it tough for quite a while. When we were at home doing the interview for *A Current Affair* a few months later, Mitchell and his girlfriend were watching Wally and me sitting there answering questions, when Wally said he'd thought of taking his life. I couldn't believe he'd said it; I couldn't believe he was that bad. I knew his depression was a concern, but considering suicide? I cried that night, I felt so helpless; and useless that I couldn't do anything for him.

I was petrified that would be the major slant of the story, especially after the reporter, Amanda Paterson, saw the reaction on my face when Wally mentioned it. I was thinking, 'No, no … you are not going to make this story about suicide. The whole story is how he's gone through epilepsy and he's coming out the other side; don't make it about suicide.' My sister couldn't watch the program because of that worry. Andrew Slack, who is a guardian angel, rang me to tell me he'd seen the finished item and not to worry, it was great. I felt relieved; and Andrew was right — Amanda did a wonderful job with the story.

When I told Wally I couldn't believe he hadn't told me he'd considered suicide, I could see the sadness in his eyes. He replied, 'But I didn't want to make you sad after what you'd already been through with John.' He was trying to protect me.

It's nine years ago now that my brother took his life; no matter how much I and others were there for him, he couldn't get himself out of that deep hole. I so wish he was able to, but we can't change that. I'm glad that Wally *was* able to. There are varying degrees of depression, just as there are with epilepsy, and different circumstances, and it doesn't discriminate; anyone at all could have to confront depression.

Of all the things Wally has done in his life, that is his biggest achievement: to come out of his post-operation depression and live his life like he is now. He's won premierships, and captained Australia, and been called the king of State of Origin, but as a human being he went beyond all that. And I am so proud of that, because it shows the personal side of Wally Lewis, not the image others see of a rugby league champion — although that special determination that is deep inside him has had a hand in both aspects of his life. I admire that in him enormously.

The strength he showed when he was feeling that low was the same strength of character that played such a part in him being a great sportsman. Jamie-Lee has inherited that. Of all the obstacles thrown her way all the time, her attitude is like, 'Well, okay; I'm just going to have to find another way to beat that one.'

Wally has come such a long way since then; he's just about the Wally Lewis of old now. As I said, he's probably a better person; better in that he's not having seizures of course, but also better in his understanding of depression and that if you do have something wrong, it isn't the end of the world. He's more aware and thoughtful; sometimes I even think he's getting a bit soft. Previously, I'd cry like a baby watching a sad movie or reading something sad and he'd say, 'What the hell are you crying for?' But I've seen a tear in his eye a few times now; he was very emotional watching the TV program on the wonderful success Peter Silburn had operating on the Brisbane girl, Bianca Saez, who had Tourette's syndrome.

There is some little window that was closed, but which has now been opened up again. Of course, there are some parts of Wally's character that are just like they were way back. Someone asked me when I knew he'd recovered and I had the old Wally back. It was the day he started ripping into me in the car. 'Why are you driving so damn slow? The lights have gone green. You can take off now ... move over and let me drive!'

I just laughed and said, 'You're back ... you're really back!'

SEVENTEEN

NOT ALONE

I WAS overwhelmed. It was such a touching experience. For almost two decades I was determined to keep my battle with epilepsy private; I saw no benefit in the wider public knowing. When that became impossible after I embarrassed myself in front of the Channel 9 cameras, I bunkered down in our home for almost a year in a very private world, except for my time in Melbourne undergoing tests and, ultimately, the operation that changed my life.

But any fear I had about what would happen once my secret slipped out was very quickly turned on its head. Here I was, sitting at our dining table, with a tear in my eye and lump in my throat as I read some of the 500 letters and cards that had been sent to me from people wishing me well with my health issues. It was truly bewildering.

I became quite emotional. For one, because so many

people had taken the time and effort to contact me. Two, that the messages came from so far and wide; well beyond the rugby league territories of Queensland and New South Wales. Thirdly, with so many of those writers being epilepsy sufferers and opening up their hearts and their lives to me in writing, I quickly realised how diverse, misunderstood and troubling the condition is in our society. I decided then and there that I'd make every effort to contact each person I could, individually, to thank them and to offer them support.

One letter in particular left a big impression on me. It came from a very brave and inspirational seven-year-old Victorian boy named Jack Fennell after he'd watched the Channel 9 interview (which I had no idea was screened in Victoria) in which I talked about my decision to go to Melbourne for my brain surgery. With Jack's and his parents' permission, I'd like to record it here:

Dear Wally,

My name is Jack Fennell and I am 7 years old. I saw you on the TV last night when you were talking about Epilepsy. I wanted you to know that I was like you and had lots and lots of seizures since I was six months old until the doctors found out that there was a problem in my brain.

I had sometimes 20–25 seizures a day. It was really hard on my Mum and Dad and brothers but really, really hard on me. I had 10½ hours surgery to get all the nasty things out of my head. It has been 2 years now and I haven't had a seizure since the operation. I was really scared but I know you will be okay like I was.

My life has changed so much. I can play on the swings and slides, ride a bike and have fun in the pool. I play football and cricket even though I am the youngest in the team. I don't really see much rugby but I have seen you play on the TV in a replay. I know you will be okay if you have the operation just like me. And I hope your nasty things in your head go away forever. You can ring me if you want and I can tell you about the hospital and what they do.

Don't be scared.

Jack Fennell

Jack's parents then added this note:

Dear Wally,

I wrote this for Jack as his writing is a bit hard to read. Jack's surgery has changed not only his life but mine and the rest of the family's. He started having seizures at six months old and continued, having them undiagnosed for five years. He would stop breathing and fall over sometimes 20 times a day. I never thought Jack would turn five, but he has. During his illness all that kept him alive was his love of sport. Golf, tennis, football and especially cricket. He has such determination that the day before surgery at Auskick he wouldn't come off the ground until he kicked a goal. He actually had a seizure on the ground and refused to come off. It was a typical Melbourne winter day, 10 degrees and pouring with rain. We let Jack stay on the ground and sure enough he took a great mark and kicked a goal from the boundary line. He then turned around to his team-mates and said, 'They can take my brain out now, I kicked a goal'.

My husband and I will never ever forget that day for the rest of our lives. Jack is an amazing kid and has a very natural talent in all sports. He was really touched by your story and wanted to let you know that if, quote, 'I can do it when I was five, Wally can do it 'cause he's old'.

Never be embarrassed because you have or had epilepsy — it needs people like you and Jack to educate society to understand the illness and get it out there. People turned their backs on us as a family when Jack was diagnosed as they were scared just as we were.

Keep your thoughts positive and good luck to you and your family.

Kathie and Jack Fennell

What an incredible boy, and wonderful family. To have 20 to 25 seizures a day! And what about refusing to leave the field before he kicked a goal? I've spoken to Kathie since, and Jack, who is now nine, still hasn't had a seizure and is becoming quite a handy cricketer — I'll follow his path with interest.

There were also letters from others who've had a full recovery from surgery similar to mine. It's just wonderful to know of the many whose lives have been changed by Gavin Fabinyi, Sam Berkovic and their staff, plus other surgeons around the country who also do an outstanding job helping those who suffer from epilepsy.

It was hard to imagine that, 17 years after I last played State of Origin, people gave me enough thought to write letters or cards; it was a very touching experience. I was just one of the many footballers who were so focused on busting our guts to be successful for our team; I was always filthy when I lost and probably wasn't the most approachable person after a match because of that. But while I, and most ex-footballers, certainly appreciated the fans and their loyalty when we were playing, I never expected it to continue as I got well into middle age. It's nice to think that my achievements touched others and, to some extent, brought happiness into people's lives when Queensland or Australia or my club teams won. To think that my 'ordeal', and the fact that so many identified with what I was going through, could touch people all these years later as well — it's very rewarding and humbling. But it should not be underestimated how so many of those people, each in their own little way, have touched me in return by their genuine warm words.

One of my favourites was a card from 92-year-old Phoebe, which reads:

I am 92 years young in March 2007. I have seen a lot of rugby league including, of course, [a lot of] Broncos matches. I love them and I write to many [players] as I was born in Murgon, Qld a long, long time ago. Without a doubt you were and still are 'Our King Wally'. With doctors and family T.L.C. you will be fine, so think positive and all the very best to you.

Phoebe & family.

To receive letters from Queensland, while appreciated, was not as unexpected as the letters I received from New South Wales — where I thought I was still 'offside'. And the fact that probably 20 per cent of the letters came from other states, including Tasmania, was so surprising; some came from New Zealand as well, and even a couple from England.

Over the years, New South Wales fans regularly let me know what they thought of me when I played for Queensland and I naturally thought I hadn't improved in their popularity ratings in the years that followed. That was evidenced by the remarks I'd cop when doing pre-match comments on the sideline for Fox Sports on their NRL coverage or Channel 9 during Origin games. So it was such an eye-opener, and remarkably comforting for me, to get messages from south of the border, basically saying, 'I hated you when you were playing but we want to wish you well in getting through your ordeal now.' And few of the notes discussed football. Mostly they were purely about health, often with mentions of people they knew who also suffered epilepsy. It's like I was a target of their attacks for the Queensland jersey I wore and the fact we had success against their heroes; that it wasn't as personal as it appeared when 'Wally's a wanker' used to be the catchcry of the Blues crowd.

Illness doesn't discriminate and perhaps my dilemma also showed the fans that I was the same as them; just as human and just as vulnerable; like I was just another bloke on the street going in the hospital because he's got something wrong with him. I'm not sure what they all felt, but what I do know is that the support from people all over Australia was the most comforting public gesture I've received in my life — and the incredible support of the Queenslanders during my playing career (and since) was overwhelming enough.

There was an email I received from a woman from Victoria who told me her husband was 61 and had been suffering epileptic fits for 40 years. He saw on the news that I'd had the surgery and been fortunate to have such a good recovery and he instantly decided he was going to do it.

He'd started having seizures shortly after they were married but, like me, insisted that no one was to know about it. After he watched the story on *ACA*, he went to Melbourne for tests and has since had an operation. He has so much quality in his life now and still hasn't had a seizure. It was just fantastic; firstly that, even at that age, he felt he had so much life to live that he wanted to do something about his quality of life; and secondly, that I could have such a profound effect on other people.

Here's part of a letter that was sent to *A Current Affair* after the item they did on me almost 12 months after the operation. It is from Heath Lindsay, who'd been diagnosed with epilepsy more than 25 years earlier:

My wife and I both sat and watched as they/you showed
the story and the actual clip of Wally Lewis having an
absence seizure when just about to present. We were both

in tears and my wife said that that was exactly what happened with me. The realisation that I was still having and had been having seizures for the past 25 years just hit me like a tonne of bricks.

I went to my doctor, who quickly referred me to a neurologist in Brisbane. This was 3 months ago. I underwent an MRI, and EEG and was put on a drug called Epilum.

I was having these absence seizures at least twice a month and now I have had none. My neurologist could not believe that I had gone untreated for 25 years and suffered all of the downside of the disease.

I have no doubt in my mind, that, if I had not seen the scene with Wally Lewis and seen the show, I would still be going through the ordeal for the NEXT 25 years too.

I guess really (with tears in my eyes even now while writing to you) I want to say Thank You Wally so much for being big enough and brave enough to share your story with the world. You changed my life and have given it a quality missing in it for so long.

Kindest Regards and much love from

Heath Lindsay

It's fairly powerful stuff when you realise the positive impact my story has had on some others. It took some time to make contact with those who left their details.

Some have slipped through the net but I've certainly spoken to hundreds of those who took time to contact me. In most cases, I've ended these conversations feeling good about life, but often quite sad too when I hear of sufferers who aren't making the progress they desire.

One such case was a young man on the Gold Coast whose mother contacted me, obviously quite exasperated at his plight. He was referred to Sam Berkovic and the team at the Austin, but during his stay he wasn't able to 'produce' seizures while the monitoring equipment was on him. They are still searching for the right path to take to help him overcome what are quite often severe seizures; despite taking nine tablets daily, he can have them six times a day. I've kept in regular contact with his mother and met the young guy who is a terrific person who deserves to have a lot better quality of life. Recently, they had contact from Queensland Epilepsy and the organisation has really helped them cope with their difficulties.

I can't help but feel a little guilty sometimes that I was suitable for, and able to have, the surgery, while others find it's not as easy as that. And I don't have the medical expertise to guide them too much other than to refer them to people who were so successful in my case. However, it doesn't guarantee that they're going to have the outcome that I am fortunate enough to enjoy.

Then there was the owner of a local menswear store close to where I live. I had known Ray Kettle for about 25 years before he confided in me one day that he'd been struggling with epilepsy and was having regular seizures. Sadly, doctors diagnosed that his struggle had been brought on by a brain tumour. After my operation, he was asking how my life was going, obviously looking for some reassurance, but as much as I wanted to help him along, I used to tell him, 'Ray, it doesn't matter what my advice is, your doctor is the best person to talk to.' I desperately wanted to help him, but he was dealing with a far greater struggle than me.

Being in charge of a large menswear fashion chain, Ray was a real workaholic and, despite his distressing battle, he refused to cut back his working hours to relieve the stress. He seemed to be getting by okay, and obviously wasn't out to seek sympathy from others as he continued his brave fight. My operation denied me the opportunity to see Ray for almost a year, and when I began getting around again I thought I'd drop in and see how he was going. When I asked one of the staff how Ray was, he said, 'Oh, mate, haven't you heard? He's passed away.' The doctors had told him he had three months to live, but sadly he lasted just four days. It hit me hard; for all the complaining I used to do, just how fortunate was I? Ray was a wonderful bloke who battled bravely until the end. I can only wish his beautiful wife Sharyn the best for the future.

It's quite bizarre how some of the letters I received reached me. Most were addressed to me at Channel 9, although some were sent to Suncorp Stadium; others were addressed to 'Wally Lewis, Queensland' or 'Wally Lewis, Brisbane'. One was very cryptic. On the front of the envelope was 'WJL', which obviously stands for Walter James Lewis, 'c/- [a nom de plume we use in the phone book]' and our address. The message read: 'Get well, mate, thinking of you. Regards [I can't make out the letters of his name/nickname].' So it's obviously someone who knows me and where I live, but I don't know who it is.

Most people were quite taken aback when I called them and said, 'G'day, it's Wally Lewis here.' I was usually met with a long pause and a suspicious 'Oh … right.' Then I'd just say, 'I received a letter from you on such and such a date,' and I could sense their brain ticking over for a few seconds before they realised, 'Oh, this must be authentic then.'

Some still didn't believe me, however. There was one bloke from NSW who had sent me a typical letter, admitting he wasn't one of my biggest fans when I was playing for Queensland but, after becoming aware of my problems, wanted to send his best wishes. I called him to say thanks but he just wouldn't accept that it was me. As soon as I said, 'This is Wally Lewis,' there was a pause and then he laughed. 'You won't get me this time, Simmo.' I said, 'Mate, I know you might think this is a gee-up — I've been a victim of a good gee-up myself from mates plenty of times — but this *is* Wally Lewis.' 'Yeah, sure, Simmo,' came the sheepish reply. I chipped in with, 'How about I leave my number and you call me back at Channel 9?' He said, 'Yeah sure, I'll call Channel 9, get through to the real Wally Lewis and make a dickhead of myself. No way in the world, Simmo.'

I then asked him whether Simmo would know he wrote me a letter. 'Well, I don't know, maybe he heard ...' I interrupted, 'Listen, fair enough. I prefer to call people to thank them for their letters, but I'll write you a letter in response and then you'll know you're not being geed up.'

Then it hit me. 'Hold on ... how about I read your letter to you now — then you'll know I'm fair dinkum.' He started to think and admitted that Simmo couldn't have got his hands on the actual letter. He paused, then I read him the opening sentence and he got all embarrassed, swore and said, 'It must be you then.'

Of course, there were bound to be those with offers of different sorts of treatments or those with quite spiritual messages. All were appreciated. I'm not a particularly religious person but I was touched when I received a few notes saying that people had prayed for me; and a couple of instances where masses were conducted in my honour. I received a note from a Baptist minister from Coffs Harbour in New South Wales, even though, when I played, he said he was barracking for the opposition. 'However, sport means little when your health is not what it should be,' he wrote. I also received a letter of best wishes from the Archbishop of Brisbane, John Bathersby.

One 'alternate' remedy came from a gentleman in New Zealand, who claimed that if I followed the attached information it would undoubtedly improve my health without the need for 'drastic surgery'. He suggested I visit a hospital that used natural methods in San Diego, California, and enclosed an article on epileptics who'd had remarkable success through increased intake of magnesium and vitamin B6. He gave a convincing argument and there is no doubt the vitamins would help, but I am glad I elected to have surgery.

I hope I'm not boring you, but here is one more letter that touched me, and gave me so much satisfaction that my story has at least raised awareness of epilepsy, and given people a clearer understanding that they may be suffering the disease.

Dear Wally,

I am writing for a few reasons, not least of which is to say THANK YOU for what you, unknowingly, have done for me.

The thank you is for this — 2 years ago today I had my first 'episode' of 'I didn't know what' — I actually thought I must be dying!!! (We always think the worst, don't we!) It has taken this past two years, many tests and two Neurologists to finally decide that my condition is part of the Epilepsy family. Because my condition doesn't actually fit into any of the 'boxes' regarding epilepsy, I (and my husband) have struggled to accept the diagnosis. However, all that changed when I saw you struggle on TV late last year and I knew immediately that my Neurologist was on the right track. It was like looking at what happens for me. If I hadn't seen what happened for you, I would no doubt still be wondering if my Neurologist had it right!

So, although this is a major trauma in your life (and that of your lovely wife and family), PLEASE take some comfort from the fact that you have helped others. I'm sure that I can't be the only one that saw you and felt as I did at the time.

At my last visit to my Neurologist a few weeks ago, and subsequently to my GP, I told each of them about this

and that I would like to write to you to say 'thank you'
and they both encouraged me to do so — so here I am.

I would also like to wish you all the very best in your
quest to find some answers to your condition and be
assured that we will keep you (and your family) in our
thoughts and prayers.

Once again, thank you, Wally (I hope it's okay to
call you Wally) for what you have done for me. I am
now moving 'upwards and onwards' (so to speak), I
hope, and have a very different outlook on how to
handle all of this.

Best wishes and I will continue to follow your case with
interest.

Kind regards,
Linda (name withheld)

I still get a lump in my throat when I read these letters
again.

While I'm expressing my appreciation of the efforts of
so many who contacted me, I can't overlook those within
the sporting community, and particularly the rugby league
fraternity. That's one valuable thing about rugby league, at
least in the era that I came through; the mateship and
camaraderie that is often regenerated when one of your
old mates needs support.

Jacqui also received constant support during my post-op period from former pro golfer Jack Newton, his wife Jackie and son Clint, who played for the Newcastle Knights and Melbourne Storm. Jack had a personal battle far greater than mine when he lost an arm, an eye and had terrible internal injuries when he walked into an aeroplane propeller in 1983 at the height of his career. The Men of League Foundation sent flowers and a nice note and I received best wishes from the National Rugby League, Australian Rugby League, Queensland Rugby League and many, many past players and officials — and of course Gene and the FOGS kept in regular contact.

After I had my operation, the Melbourne Storm sent flowers and their coach Craig Bellamy made contact with Jacqui to tell her the players would like to come around to visit me in hospital. Jacqui told them I wasn't up to seeing anyone, but a week later I thought, 'If it's good enough for them to make an effort, it's good enough for me' and I arranged to go to their training. Unfortunately, as I mentioned earlier in this book, a newspaper camera just happened to be there to turn a private visit into a public one.

I still receive probably an average of one to two calls a week at Channel 9, plus two or three letters; many from people who don't put their address on the back of the envelope so I can't reply.

Compared to the daily battles of others, I'm very fortunate. Young Jack suffered 20 to 25 seizures a day; others would have six to eight grand mals a day and are on maximum medication. I often wondered what possible comfort could they get living like that; their whole lives would be spent in fear of when the next one was coming. But after speaking to so many sufferers and their family members, I also realised that, generally, they don't tend to panic; while their parents, children, siblings etc are in constant fear, for the sufferers it's almost like, 'Oh well, it's just another one.'

I admire their courage and resilience. Although I never profess to have all the answers and always encourage them to get the right medical help, I enjoy trying to be of some comfort to them because I know it can be lonely attempting to fight that battle by yourself.

I now realise I was wrong to do that for so long.

ANOTHER PERSPECTIVE

By Helen Whitehead, CEO Epilepsy Queensland

Just after 6pm, sitting at my desk at Epilepsy Queensland. In an instant our phones went berserk.

Every line was taken with incoming calls. I learned quickly that Nine News had broken the story of Wally's epilepsy. The calls flooded our phone lines for a long time after that.

The intensity of emotion experienced by the callers was overwhelming — men sobbing, choked up, '… but Wally's the King — how could this happen?'; 'he's given so much to football/Queensland/the community — this is so unfair'; 'can you tell Wally our family is praying for him …'

We are used to helping people in distress, but normally it's a family member or the person with epilepsy that we're counselling, not people concerned about someone they only knew as a sporting and media legend. People were desperate to understand what was happening to Wally and were deeply concerned for his welfare.

Epilepsy is a condition that struggles to attract community support. Nowhere is this more obvious than in the media. I was once told 'doing a story about epilepsy would be as exciting as watching paint dry'. All this changed after Wally's story became public — I had media ringing day and night wanting to find out about Wally and epilepsy. I was more than happy to talk with them about epilepsy, but what they wanted was news of Wally.

Our hearts went out to Wally and his family. You need time and space to prepare for and recover from neurosurgery. Life would have been difficult enough without the intense public and media speculation.

Most people with epilepsy aren't suitable candidates for surgery and rely on medication for seizure control. Wally was fortunate that surgery was an option for him, although it's never a decision to be taken lightly. Queensland doesn't yet have a Comprehensive Epilepsy Service. While some patients have epilepsy surgery in Brisbane, most still have to travel to Melbourne to obtain the comprehensive care that's required. The long stay away from home is an additional burden on the family at a time when they least need it. Wally has reached out to support others contemplating surgery. You can't beat the feeling of shared experience when you're facing such a daunting time.

Wally's open admission about his epilepsy has been a turning point for other Australians with epilepsy. To know that a man of his calibre, who has achieved so much in sport and media, has faced many of the same fears, uncertainty, and difficulties associated with epilepsy, has made a difference for countless people. We now have a very powerful role model. Wally demonstrated considerable courage in stepping out of the shadows to share his story. He's given hope to many people with epilepsy and inspired them to talk about their epilepsy when, in some cases, they'd been hiding it for a lifetime. One man told me, 'God bless Wally — he will never know how much his "coming out" to talk about epilepsy has changed my life.'

Epilepsy comes in many different forms. It is not uncommon, especially with the nonconvulsive seizure types, for people not to know that they are experiencing seizures. They have a sense that something is not right but unless they are fortunate enough to have a seizure in front of a trained observer, they may go on for years without a diagnosis and the appropriate treatment. With Wally talking so openly about his seizures, it's helped individuals to get the medical attention that they need, and with it a major improvement in quality of life.

Whichever way you look at it, Wally's a great ambassador for our cause; a hero on and off the field. He's a generous man who has positively touched the lives of many struggling with the challenges of epilepsy. He has already made a significant contribution for which Epilepsy Queensland and, nationally, Epilepsy Australia will always be grateful. The Flame, our logo that symbolises enlightenment, burns brighter in Wally's presence.

One more step out of the shadows.

For information and support relating to epilepsy, please call your state's Epilepsy Australia organisation on 1300 852 853.

EIGHTEEN

CELEBRATION

I WAS confused at first. Then, when I realised it was me
the crowd was cheering — in Sydney of all places — I
got a little choked up. It was a gesture I very, very much
appreciated; and will never forget.

It was the night of the Centenary rugby league Test
match on 9 May 2008. The game was played 100 years to
the day after the first Test staged in Australia, also against
New Zealand. To celebrate the code's 100th birthday, the
Team of the Century, the 17 best players chosen from the
game's history, was announced to the crowd before the
match. I had the unbelievable honour of being chosen as
the five-eighth. The halfback was Andrew Johns and we
were to be taken around the ground on the back of a
convertible and introduced to the crowd.

The Sydney Cricket Ground had last hosted a league
Test in 1986, when I was fortunate enough to be the

Australian captain for the second Test against the Kiwis. When it came to crowd interaction, the SCG didn't hold many great memories for me. I was the number one public enemy from Queensland during my playing days and was used to boos and 'Wally's a wanker' chants (or the equally creative 'Wally sucks') when I played for the Maroons. On one occasion at the ground, the first Test of 1984, I was booed when my face came up on the big screen while the national anthem played, something that disappointed even some of the Sydney media who thought it was over the top. To be honest, I got used to it whenever I played in Sydney, and used it as motivation to perform better.

On the night of the 2008 Test match, the Team of the Century players or their representatives gathered in the Members Stand and were told the routine: we'd be introduced to the crowd, then walk onto the field, hop into the cars and slowly go around the ground. I thought, 'Here we go again. I'm going to cop a hammering when I get introduced, but don't worry about it.' I just expected it — it's the way it had always been at the Cricket Ground, so it would naturally continue.

I said to 'Joey' before we walked out, 'If we sit in the car together, at least they won't be able to boo me because everyone would think they were booing you. But to be on the safe side, how about you sit on the outside, so if any cans are thrown they'll hit you first.'

He said, 'I wouldn't be too sure it won't be me they'd be booing.' He'd come through his well-publicised drug confessions the year before and there was some debate whether he should have been picked in the Team of the Century. My view was that he should have been judged for his football, nothing else.

Anyway, we were introduced over the PA system and there was a mighty cheer. I just assumed it was for Joey as, with the echo from the speakers, I couldn't make out what was being said. I got into the car and Joey joined me a few seconds later. As we went around the ground waving to the crowd, we received really warm applause which we both appreciated greatly.

When we finished our lap someone said to me, 'I bet that's the loudest cheer you've ever received at the SCG,' and explained that the big roar I thought was for Joey was actually for me. I was a bit taken aback. It made a very special night even more special. It was just a breathtaking moment to be able to stand there in the company of the other guys like Reg Gasnier, Graeme Langlands, John Raper, Mal Meninga, Norm Provan and Noel Kelly. And what made it even more emotional was that the Coach of the Century, Jack Gibson, had passed away only a few hours before and the news was broken to the crowd.

The function at which the Team of the Century had been announced a couple of months earlier was also an incredible night, and was the first official function I attended after my operation. I still had a bit of an issue with my confidence and I'd been careful not to do any public appearances or functions where I thought I might feel a little uncomfortable. But it was just a wonderful nostalgic evening at the Hordern Pavilion, next door to the SCG; I'd never seen such a gathering of rugby league legends in the one place at the one time.

The top 100 players of the century had been chosen and they, or their representatives, were invited to the black tie dinner. It was great to take Jacqui down and catch up with so many people I'd met through the game. We gathered at the hotel across the road from the function centre and then went over to the Hordern where the 100 players were brought on stage and introduced to the audience. The most moving part of the night was when all the players had to gather backstage before being introduced to the audience. Every time I turned around I thought, 'Geez, there's such and such.' So many of them were players my old man used to tell me about; it really was a stunning moment and you could feel the pride of every single bloke who was there.

We all knew that to be chosen in that company was an enormous honour.

I'll never forget Noel Kelly, who was a Queensland legend from Ipswich and the only front-rower to make three Kangaroo tours (he toured as a hooker in 1959–60 and 1963–64 and a prop a third time in 1967–68), saying something like, 'I don't give a stuff if I make the Team of the Century, as long as they don't put me finishing last among the candidates; what a great honour just to be in the company of these blokes.' I'd heard about how tough 'Ned' was and he's a tremendously humble person; it was great to rub shoulders with him and others of his era. Another thing at those gatherings is that you realised a lot of the feared forwards of earlier days weren't all that big. John Sattler was there and I remember seeing how strongly built he was when I watched him play on TV; he's obviously lost weight since his playing days but he was a front-rower who wouldn't be as tall as me.

It was a magic night and to be chosen five-eighth in the Team of the Century was a bit of a surprise. Bob Fulton was one of the original four Immortals and could have been selected at centre or pivot, and there were other players like Vic Hey, Brad Fittler, Laurie Daley, Arthur Summons and Brett Kenny who could have been chosen at five-eighth. I was naturally very nervous, and a little emotional, when I had to get up on stage.

No matter what you achieve in your career, players always have this sense of awe about their heroes who played before them. When you're growing up you hear about these legends who created the history of rugby league; you watched or read about them and dreamed of being like them. If you were lucky enough to get the opportunity to follow in their footsteps, you'd hope to be able to reward the people who selected you, and pay respects to those before you, by living up to the standard that these legends of the game had shown. I'm sure every player in the current generation still goes through that.

I'd thought I was just a club footballer; then one day someone in the press mentioned that I might be a candidate for a spot in the Brisbane team and I was so excited. Later I was mentioned as a possible Queensland player. You never start out with those expectations. When I was chosen to play for Australia for the first time in 1981 against France, what struck me was the fact I'd taken on the responsibility of joining the tradition set by all of those names I held in such awe. Over a quarter of a century later I still feel the same about all those players, and to be in the presence of so many on the same night was incredible.

Later in the year there was a similar large function put on by the Queensland Rugby League at the Brisbane Exhibition Centre when it announced the Queensland Team of the Century. Again, to see and meet so many Queensland legends was a real honour. An even bigger honour was being chosen as captain of the team. I just feel very fortunate to have been given the opportunity to play at the level I did and to experience nights like that. The players were given replicas of the caps players were awarded back in the early 1900s when they were chosen in rep teams, but our heads were all too large in size; it was quite amusing trying to put them on.

Like so many thousands of boys, I fell into rugby league — well, I was probably born into it, considering the strong links on both sides of my family. I can still vividly remember going to my grandparents' homes, which were both within 300 metres of Lang Park. I'd take off down the road, jump the rickety old fence at the stadium and kick the ball around a playing field that was every Brisbane boy's dream to play on one day.

Obviously, the game has changed a fair bit since those times, but one thing that fortunately hasn't changed much in the last couple of decades is State of Origin. Ron McAuliffe must be sitting back in his rocking chair up in the heavens feeling pretty comfortable with what has happened to Origin football. The interest in the interstate series between Queensland and New South Wales was just about dead and buried until he campaigned for Queenslanders to be allowed to play for their home state in 1980. And we have to pay credit to the NSW Rugby League boss Kevin Humphreys, who decided it had to be experimented with when most NSW clubs and officials thought it would be a waste of time.

Nobody should ever underestimate the role Arthur Beetson played in making sure Origin football was treated seriously too. For Artie to play like he did in his only game for Queensland, aged 35 years and 167 days, is one of the most extraordinary sporting achievements that anyone has performed; you're supposed to be preparing to be a grandfather at that age! And he played the whole 80 minutes of that match (Queensland didn't use a reserve). As a 20-year-old who idolised him, I just didn't want to let 'Bean Bag' down. That night, I watched him have four blokes on him in a tackle and still slip the ball away, regularly.

I feel extremely proud that I played in that game, and had a role in establishing what State of Origin has become today. It is an international event, with people lining up to get into bars in the USA and the UK to watch a game. When I talk to athletes from other sports, they are all in awe of the intensity and quality of Origin football, no matter what sport they're involved in; they're amazed at the pace and intensity the players can achieve for 80 minutes. Just about all of them won't miss an Origin match, so it transcends well beyond just rugby league.

And although few of the current Origin players were even born when we were establishing State of Origin as a format to be taken seriously in the '80s, I think they understand the commitment required to live up to the standards that have been set in the past. That's a big reason why we see so many great games of tough, intense football. The benchmark was set early and players today know they are quite capable of taking standards to a new level each year. Origin representatives have to reach such a high level of performance in club football to be selected, and when they get there they know it is the single greatest challenge facing them.

And as a former Maroons player I was naturally extremely proud of the performances of the Queensland side in winning four straight series under Mal Meninga's coaching from 2006 to 2009. Considering that the pool of players Queensland has to pick from in the NRL is about one-third of New South Wales' and critics from the south were writing the Maroons off after losing the 2005 series, their effort to win the next four series has been outstanding. The performances of players like Adam Mogg, Steven Bell, Nate Myles, Dallas Johnston and Greg Inglis, who made such great debuts in 2006, typified the tradition that was built when blokes like Chris Close, Gene Miles, Colin Scott, Rohan Hancock, Greg Conescu, Bryan Niebling and Greg Dowling came through as young 'unknowns' — to the NSW public and media, anyway — in the pioneering years of Origin.

Before the Origin concept was born in 1980, we used to go to Lang Park as teenagers with some hope that the Queensland team would pull off an upset victory. They'd be in the match with NSW with 10 or 15 minutes to go, only to be beaten by about 20. It was our dream to one day play first grade in Brisbane — you were the bee's knees if you did that. To go one level higher and play for Queensland; well, that was just as great as it got. When that time arrived, I'd run out onto Lang Park, look into the outer at all the people and remember when I was one of them praying that Queensland would knock those bastards from the south off just once. It would take only one look at those faces, and to hear their chanting, to remind me of how important it was to represent them well. You weren't just playing for yourself and your team-mates and your coach, you were carrying everybody's hopes, and that lifted your own expectations of yourself. I felt so determined not to let them, or myself, down, and I would be filthy for a fortnight if I lost.

Nearly 30 years into State of Origin, I'm sure that feeling still exists today; despite the fact that all the Queensland representatives play in the National Rugby League, not the local Brisbane competition. Mal's insistence that contributors from past Origin campaigns play such a big role in ensuring the current players understand those traditions and those times is, I think, just wonderful. If they feel how I still feel today when I see my heroes from when I was growing up, it can only help give them an edge.

I don't think the magnitude of Queensland winning an Origin series is fully understood, considering that, as I've mentioned, they have one-third of the number of NRL players to pick from compared to NSW and that 11 of the 15 Australian NRL clubs are located in New South Wales and Canberra, and only three in Queensland. It's like Canada beating the United States; that's how I look at it.

Naturally I have some regrets when I look back on my playing career: being ruled out of the 1990 Kangaroo tour when I know I was fit; not being given the opportunity to finish my career with the Broncos; a run of injuries in my last few seasons. But, generally, I couldn't have asked for much more than what I was fortunate to have achieved.

Another regret I have to admit to is my lack of success as a coach. If I could have my time over again, I would have had a couple of years out of the game before beginning coaching. A couple of people certainly advised me that a coach should never start with a team whose players he had a close relationship with when he played. My first experience was as captain–coach of Wynnum Manly in 1986 and fortunately we won the competition; but I then had to contend with being captain–coach at the Gold Coast in 1992, then to coach the guys I played with the next year.

In 1993 and 1994 I took on the Maroons' coaching job after just one season out of the Queensland team, and I had a lot of players in the team who I'd played with; and that undoubtedly made my job more difficult. I was too close to too many of them and, for example, if I tried to get serious Allan Langer would break the mood with a 'Well, aren't *you* serious?' type of comment.

Having success as a player can also often make it harder to have success as a coach. There is always a semblance of: 'Why can't they see or do what I did?', plus you also find it harder when the team isn't performing up to the standards you enjoyed as a player. Watching the game from the sideline is easy for spectators, but the ability to assess a situation and then act upon it is far tougher for players. And ensuring it is the correct option is another demand altogether.

The other aspect of my coaching that I would have changed most, and learned a lot from, is that each player needs to be treated individually, as they respond differently to different methods. Some players perform well when the coach raises his voice in the dressing room, while for others that might be the worst thing possible.

There was once a time when coaches would treat the team as a whole, but these days there is more science and individuality to get the best out of players. A classic example I came across was Dale Shearer, one of the most naturally gifted players to have represented Queensland in Origin, who was so laidback and in his own world at times that he would not respond to the big spray or over-information. I never needed motivating and was a terrible loser; so I definitely wouldn't have been able to understand the common post-match term used today: 'We just didn't have our heads on tonight.' But I also appreciate now that all players are different and thus the big stick treatment is not always appropriate.

Generally though, as a coach, maybe I put pressure on myself to succeed too early. I look at Wayne Bennett's coaching record and all the success he has had, but it took him a while to taste success. It's all about experience, and learning from that experience over a period of years, and I didn't have the chance to get the benefit of that; I was thrust into it prematurely. I didn't have the opportunity for a natural coaching apprenticeship; instead, I took on a struggling Gold Coast Seagulls first grade side in my last season as a player and first season as a non-player, and then Queensland in the next two years after that. And there was such an internal bun fight going on at the Seagulls that enjoying the position wasn't an option.

Rugby league has always been important to me, and will continue to be. When I look back on my career in the sport, I feel very privileged and very proud to have been given the opportunity to achieve the things that I have.

I hate losing, so I have to be honest and say it doesn't sit well with me that Gold Coast came last in my two years there and Queensland lost both Origin series 2–1 when I coached. But, with Jamie-Lee's issue and my epilepsy starting to deteriorate in that period, I quickly decided there were more important things in life than football.

Learning that Jamie-Lee was deaf when she was 11 months old, and I was 31, was the first example of that. I've attended countless fundraising functions since, trying to help people who've been dealt a bit of an unfair hand with their lives, and that has opened my eyes. Then, when I had to overcome my own health issues, I further realised there are plenty of things more important in life than sport. Don't get me wrong, though: I am damn glad I've had an association with rugby league; I think sport is very important in teaching our youth some of the great attributes required to be successful in life — discipline, teamwork, physical fitness, responsibility, goal setting and overcoming adversity.

And for me, and many others, being successful in sport has given us financial advantages, even though that wasn't a motivating factor. Today, high-level sport is a full-time job — in rugby league, rugby union, soccer, AFL, cricket and a lot of sports that were regarded as 'amateur' until the past decade. I'm sure financial motivation is a much bigger part of rugby league players' make-ups these days. It is a different game in many aspects; but I still love it.

And I enjoyed being reconnected with it, to an extent, during its centenary year of 2008; at an appropriate time in my life, when I was just getting my confidence back in mixing with people and was starting to move forward as a more relaxed person, without having to deal with the fear of seizures. I felt fortunate, and very humble, being part of its festivities.

ANOTHER PERSPECTIVE

By Steve Haddan, Channel 9 Brisbane sports reporter

When Wally arrived at Channel 9, we were delighted to have the King in our midst. To tell people I worked with Wally Lewis was done with genuine pride.

Everyone asked what he was like. I'd known him socially for some years — my work as a stand-up comic had seen us meet from time to time around the footy clubs, and I always enjoyed (and was in awe of) his company. We'd once lived around the corner from each other in Norman Park in Brisbane's eastern suburbs. I thought he was a good bloke, but beyond that there was always his presence as one of the greatest league players I'd ever seen.

However, when he began working at Nine it was clear that something was not right; however, the exact nature of his condition was never revealed to me — either by Wally or those at the station who knew — until he was off to Melbourne for his surgery. I loved sharing an office with him and relished his wonderful anecdotes about players and incidents. But you could tell he was quite withdrawn, sedated, quiet, shy, slow to complete his tasks and carried with him a bottle containing a multitude of medications, which aroused my curiosity. He was reluctant to answer his phone at work and when he did he mostly mumbled and whispered to the people on the other end. I put this down to the fact that after years and years of being pestered by people, he'd simply had enough.

While all of his colleagues gladly and willingly helped where we could, I often wondered what was going on; but I was determined not to stick my nose in. As the father of an epilepsy patient — my late son Freddie — knowing what he was going through would have made everything a whole lot easier. To later learn he had battled the condition since the age of 20 was astonishing. The challenge of keeping this bottled up inside him must have been immense.

The pressure he was under was clear. When he had his turns while reading the bulletin on air you could feel the pain he was going through. When he stumbled his way through live crosses and struggled as a special comments man during live broadcasts, I felt genuinely sorry for him. But while the secret remained largely a closed shop, the view that he was just another footballer who'd had too many hits to the head was allowed to prevail. People would ask me what was wrong with Wally; I'd simply reply I didn't know.

When he returned to work following his recovery from successful brain surgery, the change in his demeanour was astonishing. He now has this spring in his step. The contrast between the withdrawn, mumbling epilepsy sufferer, exposed to the humiliation of on-air gaffes which no one understood, and the outgoing, cheerful, enthusiastic person he's become is remarkable. To see him relishing and negotiating his on-air tasks with all the gusto you'd expect from the game's greatest player is bringing genuine happiness to all who work with him. Let's face it — no rugby league coverage is complete without Wally's two bob's worth!

Wally is the only bloke here at the Channel 9 sports desk who gets any fan mail! During his recovery, he'd get dozens of letters a day which piled up on his desk in his absence. When he returned to his desk he spent months working his way through literally hundreds of letters, writing back, and when the folk left phone numbers, Wally would call and spend hours talking to them. Knowing the difficulties epilepsy patients and their families suffer — the misconceptions, the fear and the stigma — I can only imagine what a call from the King would have done.

When he'd say it was Wally Lewis calling, none of them believed him! He was all class. His doctors worked a miracle with Wally and we are all delighted he's made a full recovery from the pain and uncertainty he's been through.

NINETEEN

A FORTUNATE LIFE

'*Sport now with Wally and there are no surprises in our Origin squad.*'

When I get the throw from the newsreader these days to preview the sport before the break, I'm usually fairly relaxed.

'*I don't think too many people were expecting them, Bruce — we'll take a look at the Maroons' Origin line-up next.*'

[Take vision of Lleyton Hewitt's winning point]

'*Lleyton Hewitt again shows he's a fighter.*'

[Take vision of Indy 500 crashes]

'*… and the Indy 500 — not for the fainthearted.*'

I'm only on camera for about 15 seconds before breaking for the commercials. I tend to breeze through that okay, but I still get nervous during the next three minutes.

The nerves are nothing like they were before, though, when I used to be petrified … of having a seizure.

'*Okay, Wal … 60 seconds 'til we're back.*'

It's still very much like when I played football; no matter how many times I'd strapped on the boots and run onto the park, I still had the pre-match nerves and the heart would start racing.

'*Thirty seconds …*'

The worst thing I feel now is, 'Did I just sense something?' It's only happened once or twice and maybe it's a subconscious thing that I'm always on guard for a possible seizure. But I quickly tell myself, 'Don't worry about it.'

Apart from that, my biggest fear when I'm on air now is, 'Don't stuff up the names. Get the pronunciations right, whatever you do, Wally.'

'*Five … four … three … two … one.*'

The finger is pointed at me and I'm on.

'*Selectors have once again placed their faith in Queensland's reigning State of Origin champions, with just one change made from last year's winning side. Skipper Darren Lockyer returns, alongside hitman Mick Crocker, who was expected to be completing his career in England.*'

After a few more items, it's over for another night.

I admit I still let out a sigh of relief to myself when I come off. It's not 'Thank Christ for that' and a wipe of the sweat from my forehead, like it used to be. It's now more of a case of: 'I'm glad that's over — I didn't seem to make any little blues tonight.'

I'll return to my office, grab my gear and, invariably, I'll have a smile on my face on my way out of the building. I'll hop in the car for the 45–50 minute trip home, feeling a lot more relaxed and reassured; knowing I'm no chance of having an 'aura' and having to pull over … and knowing Jacqui isn't worried sick about me getting home safely. But it's still the same drive, the same route, the same routine.

When I walk in the door, that's when my new life feels a lot different. I don't have this overpowering need to slump in the lounge chair and 'veg out'. The rest of the family don't give me a wide berth, knowing I need some time to come good. In fact, most nights when I get home I'll say hello, sit on the kitchen bench and get harangued by Jacqueline to take my work clothes off before hopping into my meal, so I don't spill food on them. Ah, life is back to normal!

I feel a lot more alert; I'll often stay up until 10pm or 10.30pm, whereas before I would often be asleep on the lounge chair by eight. I can have a conversation with Jacqui or one of the kids, and watch a television program at night and see the end of it.

If a social invitation arrives, I'm more likely to accept it; no longer having to make an excuse because of my complete lack of confidence when talking to anyone except the family and close friends. I am much more comfortable in groups, and with old friends who I'd almost cut myself off from. Brian Ball, Peter Gamble, Allan Mohle, Mark Wilson and I play tennis one night a week which I find enjoyable and entertaining, as it often is with such good old mates who like to take the piss out of each other at every opportunity. I would have been too tired, and too uncomfortable, to do that before the operation.

Jacqui would say I am a better person now than I ever was before. I'm more considerate and aware of others, more patient, more tolerant and more compassionate. Certainly, I am more comfortable with the person I am.

Perhaps my ordeal was a reward, in a strange sense. While I didn't enjoy the trauma it created for my family at the time, the success of the temporal lobectomy surgery has enabled me to appreciate life more and has motivated me to become an advocate for awareness of epilepsy. It is a disease so few people know enough about, even someone who suffers it like me; and we have to change that.

I am in such awe of how Sam Berkovic, Gavin Fabinyi and others at the Austin Medical Centre enriched my life that I'm now motivated to ensure I assist families and others who suffer epilepsy with any encouragement I can give them. To be able to speak to families who have the difficulty of having a sufferer around them is very rewarding, although it can be difficult at times.

When I get on the phone and hear a mother cry her eyes out, and then speak to the father who is usually less emotional but equally supportive of their child, I get quite choked up as well. And I am not naturally an emotional person.

I was at Channel 9 recently and had just finished a phone conversation with a fellow sufferer who'd contacted me, when my colleague Steve Haddan said, 'You get a buzz out of doing that, don't you?' Before I could answer yes, he said, 'You're spending hours on the phone every week and you obviously really enjoy it; I think it's terrific.' I broke the mood up before I got involved in explaining my feelings too deeply with, 'Yeah, if Lee [Anderson] finds out how much my phone bill is going to be, he mightn't be too happy though.' But when I stopped to think about it, I do enjoy it, and get a lot of satisfaction out of it.

I still haven't had a seizure since my operation. I am feeling confident I never will, although no one can guarantee you're 100 per cent immune to that happening. At my two-year check-up in late February 2009 I was hoping to get a more excited response from the medicos. Dr Berkovic and Dr O'Shea were very matter of fact about where I was and it was a case of: 'So far, so good — see you next time.' I was expecting some sort of celebration; I felt like breaking out the champagne, because I'd reached what was the stated benchmark of what could be determined as a complete recovery — the two-year mark. But doctors have to be conservative; and there can never be any assurances. A classic example of that came from a woman who rang to talk about forming an information website for former epilepsy sufferers and those in post-operative stages. She declared it had been seven years since her operation, and while she still hadn't had a seizure, she was still visiting Sam and the team in Melbourne for annual check-ups.

My daily dosage of medication has been greatly reduced. I take three-and-a-half Tegretol 200 milligram tablets a day (two in the morning and one and a half in the evening), while the Dilantin has been reduced to just one 100 milligram tablet a day. While I'm also still taking half of a Cipramil 20 milligram tablet to keep depression in check, I'm hoping to eliminate that soon.

Helen Whitehead, the CEO of Epilepsy Queensland, contacted me back in 2007 and I told her that, when I felt I'd recovered well enough from the operation, I'd be happy to help her organisation's quest to raise awareness. I have assisted with some of their fundraisers and we took part in a television awareness campaign; if it has to do with switching on the light about epilepsy, I'm keen to help. I'll also continue to assist in raising funds for the Austin Hospital's epilepsy program where I can and I enjoy talking individually to sufferers or their families, if I feel I can help.

I'm still devoted to assisting in fundraising and awareness for the Hear and Say Centre in Brisbane, which had such a positive impact on Jamie-Lee's and our family's lives. They also now have centres on the Gold Coast, Sunshine Coast, Townsville and Toowoomba and an outreach program for rural and remote children. It is a charity-based organisation that does a wonderful job, with its paediatric auditory-verbal and cochlear implant techniques.

On the rugby league front, I also enjoy being involved with the Queensland FOGS program which is doing a good job in the indigenous community, with mentor schemes that are having positive outcomes in encouraging indigenous youth in their schooling and getting jobs.

I'm also enjoying being part of Channel 9's *Friday Night Football* team and Sunday coverage; my passion for rugby league hasn't waned in the least.

I'm watching Jamie-Lee grow into a young, independent woman who has achieved remarkable success by being included in Australian water polo teams; seeing Lincoln live his dreams on television and Mitchell work hard to chase his career goals (too hard, I sometimes tell him), and I do all that with more energy; taking in a lot more and being more involved.

Jacqui can live a life where she is more than a nurse-maid to an ill husband, and mother and father to our three wonderful children, and we do a lot more together. And now I've got the energy to answer her back when she nags me!

My short-term memory is still not the best, but it doesn't frustrate me like it used to. I have finally accepted that as one shortfall I am stuck with, but that is an extremely small price to pay for my improved health.

I'm looking forward to the rest of my life being as normal as possible. I enjoy being myself again and taking part in the things that entertained me for so long. And I hope I can be some sort of example, an inspiration perhaps, for others to confront their epilepsy more quickly and more openly than I did. Many have far more severe and frequent seizures and auras than I did, and have had their lives affected a lot more seriously, and I can imagine how difficult that is. Not everyone can have the happy ending that I have had; and that is the hard thing for me to accept as I talk to people who haven't been able to undergo the surgery. But many can, and have, while others can get wonderful help and support to improve the quality of their lives.

As I said early in the book, epilepsy is a battle; a tough one at that. But it need not be a sentence. To those who ensured it wasn't for me, I owe my current wonderful life.

For most people, a new day begins at sun-up or sometime after. For me, another bright day begins around 6.20pm every evening.

'Sixty seconds, Wally …'

The evening countdown no longer holds any fear.

Thank you, Sam. Thank you, Gavin.

EPILOGUE

I WAS sitting on the plane on the way back from Melbourne where I had visited the place that I'm so familiar with now, the Austin Medical Centre, and thought to myself, 'That's the most comforting, reassuring year I have had for a long, long while.' I'd been given the 'three-year; all-clear' judgement by Sam Berkovic and was pretty damn happy, as expected as the positive verdict was.

I can remember a few people saying to me after I'd had my first yearly check-up since I'd had the surgery that, 'Gee, that year has gone quick,' and I was left thinking, 'You have to be kidding; not from where I have been sitting (and I'd done a lot of sitting).' The time had dragged, with so much waiting and wondering whether I was ever going to be my old self again. The next year was better, as I started to sense light at the end of the tunnel and the anxiety about having seizures again had diminished while, socially, I was gradually reacquainting myself with old friends and old activities.

But the next year whistled past. I'd hit the half-century mark so I was officially 'old' and had a wonderful party to celebrate. I'd cut my medication right down; enjoyed my role advocating epilepsy awareness in an advertising campaign and fundraisers for Epilepsy Queensland and felt I'd really taken large steps forward with my health, fitness and confidence. And I'd received nothing but positive feedback from the release of this book, which prompted a bit of a flurry of calls, emails and letters from people who had also been affected by epilepsy; people I was generally happy to encourage and share stories with as I became more and more aware of a growing feeling within us that sharing our experiences and 'coming out of the cupboard' was now fine to do. The stigma is being beaten.

And I'd hit the benchmark of three years without a seizure since having the operation.

The thing that I still find rather startling is the amount of people, many whom I'd known for a long while, who have confided in me that they have someone in their family who suffers from the condition. One example came during a golf day held by the Men of League Foundation, which assists retired footballers. A mate I'd known during my early footy days in Brisbane started talking about his daughter who'd had a tough time with epilepsy. I told him, 'Mate, I had no idea,' and he said, 'No, she has been dealing with it for some time now but we don't tell people about it; we see no need to promote the fact she's an epileptic; we just prefer for her to deal with it privately.'

But we all need support, understanding and education. That's why I was happy to appear in Epilepsy Queensland's television and radio advertising campaign which was launched in late 2009. It starts with me saying, 'I had epilepsy and I'm happy to talk about it because an epileptic seizure is just a break in … [sounds starts to break up] break in … transmission.' A graphic comes on the screen [someone speaks the words in the radio version] saying, 'We apologise for this break in transmission. One in 50 people have these interruptions. To find out how to help them through a seizure, go to www.epilepsyqueensland.com.au.' Then it goes back to me finishing off the sentence, 'To make sure you know how to help them through a seizure. And if the people around me know what to do, I know I'm okay.'

I think it's a terrific analogy to show how people feel when they suffer an epileptic seizure; certainly that was the case for me — I would virtually go 'off the air' for those few seconds.

So, generally, life is good. I'm enjoying work at Channel 9 and I'm into my second season on the National Rugby League commentary team, going to two matches most weekends. I'm still playing tennis with the boys when I get a chance and get out on the golf course at every opportunity, usually for an organised event, and get real satisfaction talking to epileptic sufferers and helping them where I can. To be honest, I think the most enjoyable moments start at home. I'm not confined to the chair in the lounge room fearful of a seizure at any unexpected moment, and every opportunity I get is spent in the back yard. I'm probably one of the few blokes who doesn't think 'knocking over the lawn' or 'washing the kids' cars' is a chore; for me it's the time spent doing the mundane things like that which make me appreciate life after I was confined in my everyday lifestyle for so long.

My medication has been reduced to just three and a half Tegretol tablets a day, while I'm down to half a Cipramil tablet a day as an anti-depressant. I'll wean down off that over the next 18 months or so. I don't have an issue still taking the anti-depressant because I know what benefit it has provided. Again, a stigma removed.

I'm one of the lucky ones. I was suitable for the surgery and it has worked. I still hear occasionally from the parents of Michael, the young chef on the Gold Coast, who are frustrated that there just doesn't seem to be any breakthrough for him; they just can't force seizures to occur when he goes in for testing and they feel as though they can't get the right help.

I keep in contact with Steve from Darwin, who shared that experience with me at the Austin when I went in for the surgery, and he is an inspiration to me as much as I might have inspired others. Steve still suffers seizures on average every couple of days but doesn't complain and doesn't feel sorry for himself. His attitude is, 'Oh well, that's the way it is; it didn't work out for me so I just get on with life, but I am really glad it has for you, Wally.' His outlook is to make the most of his life, despite the disappointment that he couldn't have the surgery to end his suffering. While I feel sad for Steve that he didn't have the outcome I did, he lifts me with his incredible spirit.

There is so much positivity around me in my family too. Jacqui, as always, is fully of beans and making the most of any hour of the day and it's great that we can do so much together again. Lincoln shot a movie in 2009, *Tomorrow: When The War Began*, based on the novel by John Marsden, and as I write this we're waiting for its release at the cinemas. He was then moving onto a role with the Channel 9 serial *Rescue Special Ops*.

Mitchell has progressed from glorified coffee boy on the breakfast show at Nova 106.9FM in Brisbane to be the sports presenter. Breakfast show hosts Meshel and Tim have tagged him 'The Prince' in a play on my moniker of 'The King' and while it gave him a giggle at first, I think it wore on him after a while. He thought one way to get them to ease off a bit was to sign off the sports news a couple of times with, 'That's the sport and I'm The Prince.' It seems to have worked! He loves the job, even with its early morning rise from bed, and he still works part time at the cinema too. I'm proud of him.

Jamie-Lee continues to do well with her water polo, with her club team the Brisbane Barracudas winning the national league competition in 2009 and, as I put this together, they're into the finals in 2010. She's now played for the Australian Schoolgirls, the Queensland and Australian under-20s squads (part of the 2009 and 2010 squads) and won the 2009 Athlete with a Disability of the Year. She was chosen as the face of the Hear and Say Centre's annual Butterfly Appeal to help raise money for the centre, which meant she had to do an address at the launch function and some radio interviews and she handled it really well. She has also been selected as the face to promote Australia's campaign for the next Deaflympics in Athens in 2013, which is effectively the

Olympic Games for athletes around the world suffering from hearing loss.

There are still some pitfalls being the only deaf girl in her teams. When she was away with the Australian under-20s, the fire alarm went off and they'd all gathered at the meeting point when someone realised Jamie-Lee wasn't there and had to go and get her. She takes the cochlea implant out when she sleeps, so she couldn't hear a thing. There's no use ordering a wake-up call for her either, so when they have early morning meetings, one of the other girls is assigned to get her up. But it hasn't held her back as far as competing and she has ambition to represent Australia at the Deaflympics and also the Olympics in the next few years.

I've been very happy with the public response to the first release of the book. The best thing is the amount of people who have come out of the cupboard and owned up to the fact they suffer from epilepsy and are now confiding with those around them. If reading my story has encouraged them to do that in any way, or just made them feel not so isolated and alone because I have revealed a similar story to theirs, then the main motivation for telling my whole story, warts and all, in the book has been realised. The start of one letter I received, from Ray Seidel of Ipswich, perhaps sums up the feelings of many: *'Wally, I have just finished reading your book 'Out of the Shadows' and would like to thank you for writing it on behalf of all epileptics. Some of us still live in the shadows, but it is nice to know some of us have made it out into the sun.'* Those sentiments are just a bonus for me and the biggest satisfaction I get from this book is knowing that epilepsy — and the struggle confronted by its sufferers — is no longer swept under the carpet and people are more comfortable admitting they are one of the many thousands affected by epilepsy; it's no longer something to be ashamed about.

I find it easy to talk to people who are struggling to deal with their situation. I'm not a doctor and can't always come up with the answers they need. But I often put down the phone or walk away from someone I have met at a function somewhere and feel extremely satisfied that I might have been able to help in just a small way; in helping them confront their problems that little bit more bravely or leaving a little better educated having talked to someone who has gone through what they have. When I talk with people who have decided to follow the surgery path it is often good that I don't hear from them for a while afterwards, which normally indicates it has been a case of 'so far, so good'.

However, epilepsy treatment and research needs more funding, and there has to be greater understanding about how it affects people, and I help where I can there. When I went to Melbourne for my three-year check-up I timed it so I could attend a fundraising golf day in Sydney for epilepsy awareness; it was organised by advertising executive Wayne Rowley (one of his children suffers epilepsy) from the company Hyperbole, which deals with the entertainment industry. I agreed to be patron for his fundraising initiative and he organised a lot of entertainers to attend; it was a great day. I played my round of golf with comedian Billy Birmingham in my group and it was the funniest day on the golf course I have ever had. If it wasn't tough enough trying to stay in play and avoid the mass of salt bush on the famous St Michael's course along the coastline, doing it with Billy within earshot was damn near impossible. I've never laughed so much on the golf course; my stomach was hurting as, for 18 holes, he didn't stop with his comments and funny commentary in a vast range of different voices; what a talent. He hit the ball very well too.

I asked Sam Berkovic if he'd mind travelling up for the day to accept a cheque. I don't think he was all that comfortable being surrounded by a host of comedians and entertainers (he's definitely not a golfer). But I think he was intrigued by the varying personalities, and dress combinations, of those who attended! Four days earlier we'd met privately while I was in Melbourne for my three-year check-up and it was certainly a different surrounding. As usual I had results of blood samples sent down previously and felt well within myself and hadn't had a hint of a seizure, so I was naturally fairly relaxed about another six-monthly consultation.

Typically, Sam was very matter-of-fact in his conversation and we went through how I was feeling, talked about alterations to my medication and agreed that my life was good. Then came the setting of our next appointment date, and Sam surprised me with, 'Now, when would you like to come back, Wally? Do you want to make it six months or not come back for 12 months?' I thought, 'That's encouraging, not having to get checked for a whole year; I'm into the second phase of recovery now.' But I understood Sam was the one to judge that, not me. 'Am I right to come back in 12 months Sam? You'd know better than me.' 'Yes ... yes, I think so ... I think 12 months would be quite fine.'

So we shook hands and I walked out into the corridor, feeling pretty damned pleased with myself. I'd come a long way and one of the most respected epilepsy specialists in the country didn't see the need to monitor me for a whole year. Just then a young woman introduced herself to me; she was hard not to notice with a nose ring in each nostril and three or four studs in each eyebrow. But she had the most softly spoken voice and was a really warm person. She hadn't had a seizure in some time but, out of the blue, had been confronted by one and it appeared that further surgery was her only option.

Straight away my mind went back to a couple of patients who had undergone the surgery who I'd come across during my visits. One woman had gone eight or nine years without a seizure and then, bang, they'd started again. Then there was the young boy from Bundaberg who was just ten days short of the two-year anniversary of his successful operation when he had a major seizure. For all of us to go back for a check-up and hear the words that everything is alright will remain the insurance for us that we're always looking for.

Just then I also saw Louise Rafter, the sister of tennis legend Pat. I'd spoken to Louise a few times as she kept seeking reassurance that she was doing the right thing by electing to have the same surgery as me. She's taken the final step and had the operation but unfortunately she was still having seizures a couple of days afterwards and even after further surgery the seizures continued. That breaks my heart; knowing how gloriously your life can change if the operation is a success but also being so aware that not everyone can get the complete relief they are after.

And as I sat on the plane from Melbourne to Brisbane and stared out across the sky the reality hit me that, as wonderful as my life had become as I entered the fourth year since Sam and Gavin turned my life around, it only takes one phone call or one person to walk through a door and tell me of their battles to bring me back to earth and remind me not to get to blasé or carried away. And it spurs me to provide whatever encouragement, comfort and understanding of their situation that I can because, well, what if I hadn't had the good fortune that I've had; what would my life be like now?

So many epileptic sufferers I speak to share that view and a warm desire to help others. Perhaps that's because always in the back of our minds that when we come across someone who is still having trouble, is the feeling of 'that could be me again one day'. There is no guarantee I won't have a seizure or series of seizures again.

If that does happen though, at least it's so comforting to know that the support system is there; and it is getting better. I will continue to play my role in getting that message across. I'm one of the fortunate ones.

FAMOUS PEOPLE WITH EPILEPSY

Bud Abbott
Alexander the Great
Alfred the Great
Aristotle
Napoleon Bonaparte
Richard Burton
Lord Byron
Julius Caesar
Lewis Carroll
Charles V of Spain
Agatha Christie
Professor Manning Clark
Leonardo Da Vinci
Charles Dickens
Danny Glover
Tony Greig
George Frideric Handel
Hannibal
Margaux Hemingway

Louis XIII of France
Martin Luther
Michelangelo
Sir Isaac Newton
Alfred Nobel
Nicolo Paganini
Paul I of Russia
Peter the Great
Edgar Allen Poe
Pythagoras
Jonty Rhodes
Theodore Roosevelt
Robert Schumann
Sir Walter Scott
Socrates
Peter Tchaikovsky
Vincent van Gogh
Hugo Weaving
Neil Young

ABOUT THE AUTHOR

NEIL CADIGAN, an Australian Sports Writer of the Year, has had seven books published in the past three years since he co-wrote the bestselling Andrew Johns autobiography *The Two of Me*, a nomination for the 2007 Australian biography of the year. He has also written the autobiography of rugby league hero Danny Buderus (*Talent Is Not Enough*), compiled *Rugby League Yarns*, a collection of humorous and incredible stories from rugby league's century-old history and previously co-wrote the life stories of footy legends Ray Price and Brett Kenny.

Outside of rugby league he has written a biography on pioneering Australian aviator Lester Brain (*Man Among Mavericks*), co-wrote *When Silver Is Gold*, the autobiography of Olympic swimmer Brooke Hanson and the incredible life story of tsunami hero Donny Paterson (*No Ordinary Bloke*).